# Assessment of Prior Learning

## A Practitioner's Guide

Malcolm Day

Published in 2002 by:
Nelson Thornes Ltd
Delta Place
27 Bath Road
CHELTENHAM
GL53 7TH
United Kingdom

02  03  04  05  06  /  10  9  8  7  6  5  4  3  2  1

A catalogue record for this book is available from the British Library

ISBN 0 7487 6933 1

Page make-up by Acorn Bookwork

Printed and bound in Spain by GraphyCems

# Contents

# ACKNOWLEDGEMENTS

I would like to acknowledge the assistance given to me by the Council for Adult and Experiential Learning (CAEL) and the South East Education Consortium (SEEC). Also my thanks to Dr Morris Keeton, University of Maryland and members of the Experience Based Education Department at Sinclair College, USA; the School of Nursing and Midwifery at the University of Natal; the Natal College of Nursing and Midwifery; the Ministry of Health, Kwa Zulu Natal, South Africa; Pauline Tweedale at the School of Nursing and Midwifery, University of Nottingham, England.

I would also like to show my appreciation to the First Nations Technical Institute, Tyendinaga Mohawk Territory, Ontario and the Canadian Association for Prior Learning Assessment (CAPLA). In particular, I am grateful for the friendship, wisdom and guidance offered to me by Deb Blower, Ron Conlon, Mark Gallupe, Diane Hill, Banakonda Kennedy, Reg Tucker, Lynn Wilson and Paul Zakos.

Finally, a very special thank you to Professor Carolyn Mann and to Dr Thembisile Khanyile. Their considerable knowledge of APL in the USA and in South Africa has made a unique contribution to this book.

*Malcolm Day*

# About the Author

Malcolm Day, M.Phil., M.Ed., B.Ed., RGN, RNT, Dip.N.(Lond.), Cert.Ed., ILTM, is Senior Nursing Lecturer at the School of Nursing and Midwifery, University of Sheffield, England, where he teaches curriculum studies to the education pathway of the Master in Medical Science Nursing Degree, and research awareness to the Bachelor in Medical Science Nursing Degree.

He has extensive experience in the field of work-based learning and competence-based assessment. He was responsible for setting up and directing the Sheffield and North Trent College and Employers National Vocational Qualifications (NVQ) Consortium. This work received a quality award from the UK Central Council for the Education and Training of Social Workers.

Malcolm is co-researcher and co-author of two National Health Service Management Executive reports: 'Utilizing national occupational standards as a complement to nursing curricula' (1995) and 'The factors which may enhance or inhibit the use of occupational standards as a complement to the continuing education of health care professionals' (1999).

In September 1996, Malcolm was awarded a British Council Professional Exchange Grant to undertake a study visit to British Columbia. In June and October of 1997, he returned as visiting scholar in competence-based assessment, and an external adviser to the assessment service at Douglas College in Vancouver.

From May 1998 until January 2000, Malcolm was seconded from Sheffield University to the Canadian Association for Prior Learning Assessment (CAPLA) and the First Nations Technical Institute (FNTI), where he was Principal Researcher to the National Canadian Benchmarking Study for Prior Learning Assessment. The results of this project were published in 1999 by Human Resources Development Canada (HRDC) and CAPLA, in three volumes.

During his secondment to CAPLA, Malcolm also worked as Chief Education Policy Adviser to the Canadian Technology Human Resources Board (CTHRB) 'Technofile' and 'Validating Agent' Project. He was responsible for designing and evaluating a workplace APL strategy for assessment of technicians and technologists within Canada. This work was published, in three volumes, by the CTHRB in the latter part of 1999.

Malcolm has published widely in the field of work-based learning and competence-based assessment. He is author of *The Role of the NVQ Assessor*, published by Nelson Thornes in 1996.

He is a Ph.D. student at the Institute for Life-Long Learning at the University of Sheffield, England. His field of study is assessment of prior learning.

Malcolm can be contacted at: m.r.day@sheffield.ac.uk

# INTRODUCTION

The author's experience of work-based and experiential learning in North America and the UK has led to an increased awareness of the relationship between accreditation frameworks and the assessment and recognition of prior learning. In the UK, experience of delivering National Vocational Qualifications (NVQs) and professional nursing diplomas and degrees has highlighted the importance of *credit exchange*, or credential-based, models of assessment of prior learning. This approach emphasizes *products*, the achievement of competencies and the accreditation of prior certificated learning, whereas, in North America, a more *developmental* approach towards assessment of prior learning is used. This approach emphasizes *process* and the assessment and accreditation of prior experiential learning, which is often derived from work and community-based experiences.

The North American preference for a more developmental approach is, in part, due to the early influence of the Council for Adult and Experiential Learning (CAEL), and the ongoing influence of the First Nations culture, particularly the work of Diane Hill at the First Nations Technical Institute in Ontario. Also, both the USA and Canada are governed by federal systems of government: there are no nationally agreed accreditation frameworks for post-compulsory education. The responsibility for ensuring currency and transferability of credentials rests with federal government bodies, while the delivery of credentials is the responsibility of state and provincial governments. The potential for mismatch is great, particularly as economic and cultural influences within each Canadian province and American state are so diverse.

A recent international study undertaken by the Canadian Association for Prior Learning Assessment (CAPLA) indicates that occupational and professional associations within North America are now showing an increased interest in the credit exchange, or credential-based, model of assessment of prior learning (Day, 2000). This is in part due to the effects of globalization and the need for occupations and professions to demonstrate that they can practise within a globally competitive market, to an internationally acceptable standard. As a consequence of this emerging interest, a more eclectic or *complementary* approach towards assessment is beginning to emerge, where the best principles of practice from developmental *and* credit exchange models are now being used to enhance the validity and reliability of assessment decisions. Similar approaches are now emerging in UK universities, for example, in schools of health care.

This text examines the factors currently influencing assessment practice, and how assessors are attempting to resolve emerging issues in order to identify a more transparent and systematic approach towards assessment of experiential learning. Throughout the text examples of assessment practice are drawn from post-compulsory and continuing adult education within Canada, the UK, South Africa and the USA.

## THE PURPOSE OF THIS BOOK

This text is intended to encourage adult education students, and newly appointed APL assessors and advisers, to purposefully apply proven assessment theory to the practice of the assessment of prior learning. It identifies and discusses the basic principles and processes necessary for the effective and systematic assessment of prior learning. These are solidly rooted in Canadian, UK and US practice, and are currently being developed within South Africa. It is hoped that the assumptions, values, beliefs and practices espoused in this text will be applied in flexible, innovative and thoughtful ways that are respectful of the diverse backgrounds, interests and needs of adult learners.

## DEFINING THE TERMS

For the purpose of this text, *assessment* is defined as:

> *whenever one person in some kind of interaction, direct or indirect, with another is conscious of obtaining and interpreting information about the knowledge and understanding or abilities and attitudes of this other person.*
>
> Rowntree (1987)

Brown *et al.* (1996) state that the purpose of assessment is to:

> *Classify or grade students;*
> *Enable student progression;*
> *Guide and improve student performance;*
> *Facilitate student's choice of options;*
> *Diagnose faults and enable students to rectify mistakes;*
> *Give teachers feedback on their teaching;*
> *Motivate students;*
> *Provide statistics for the course, or for the institution; and*
> *Add variety to students' learning experience and add direction to teaching and instruction.*

Some of these activities are *diagnostic* as: 'they provide an indicator of the learner's aptitude and preparedness for a programme of study and identify possible learning problems' (QAA, 2000: 4), for example, to facilitate a student's choice of options. Other assessment activities may be *formative* as they are: 'designed to provide learners with feedback on progress and inform development, but do not contribute towards the overall assessment' (QAA, 2000: 4), for example, to guide and improve a student's performance.

Diagnostic and *formative* assessment activities are learner-focused or client-directed, as they are directly concerned with meeting the learner's needs. Other assessment activities may be terminal or *summative* as they: 'provide a measure of achievement or failure made in respect of a learner's performance in relation to the intended learning outcomes of the programme of study.' (QAA, 2000: 4), for example, to classify or grade students. Summative assessment activities are organizationally-focused as they are arranged to meet the demands and requirements of the educational institution.

*Assessment of prior learning* (APL) is defined as a systematic process that involves the identification, documentation, assessment and recognition of learning (i.e. skills, knowledge and values). This learning may be acquired through formal and informal study including work and life experience, training, independent study, volunteer work, travel, and hobbies and family experiences. Recognition of prior learning can be used toward the requirements of education and training programmes, occupational and/or professional certification, labour market entry, and organizational and human resource capacity building (Day, 2000).

One of the difficulties encountered in trying to understand assessment of prior learning is the range of acronyms that are often used by different people, and in different countries. For example, in the United States it is known as *prior learning assessment* or PLA (Keeton, 2000). In Canada, it is known as *prior learning assessment and recognition* or PLAR (Blower, 2000). In South Africa and Australia, it is known as *recognition of prior learning* or RPL (Flowers and Hawke, 2000; Harris, 2000). In the UK, it is known as AP(E)L. This term is generally used as an all-encompassing term to include prior *certificated* learning, as well as prior *experiential* learning (SEEC, 1995).

Within the UK, AP(E)L includes:

- *accreditation of prior achievements* (APA) – the claimant exchanges proof of past achievements in the workplace for unit credits within a nationally-agreed framework (Simosko, 1992)
- *accreditation of prior certificated learning* (APCL) – learning for which certification has been awarded by an educational institution or another education or training provider
- *accreditation of prior experiential learning* (APEL) – uncertificated learning gained from experience.

Within this text, the term *assessment of prior learning* will be used as a definition to encompass all of the above terms, and the acronym *APL* will be used with this specific meaning in mind.

For the purpose of this text, an *APL practitioner* is defined as an individual who utilizes learner-focused activities to diagnose and formatively or summatively assess an individual's prior learning, either for academic credit or recognition of competence, using the goals and methods outlined above. This definition includes the work of the *APL adviser* and also the work of the *APL assessor*, who is often but not exclusively a subject-matter expert from faculty. It may aso include the work of the *APL co-ordinator*, if he or she is directly involved in the guidance and assessment of individual candidates, or groups of candidates.

Also in this text, assessment of prior learning has been differentiated from the process of *accreditation* or *recognition* of prior learning as it is the practice of prior learning *assessment* which is the focus of this publication. The methods that might be used to assess prior learning include assessment of educational documents, portfolio review, demonstration or challenge processes (e.g. written/ oral examinations, projects, assignments, performance observation, skill demonstrations, simulations and product assessments), standardized tests and programme review.

## THE CONTENTS OF THIS BOOK

- Chapter 1 is based on the UK experience. It describes the concept of APL and its theoretical underpinnings. It discusses the potential benefit of APL to learners, employers and education institutions. It also describes the relationship of APL to the establishment of a credit-based system for the curriculum, and the factors which might influence the development of this. Finally, this chapter identifies emerging benchmarks for practice, and how these are being used to resolve issues currently influencing the APL process.
- Chapter 2 describes the experience of APL from an international perspective. Contributions are made from experts in the field including Professor Carolyn Mann who is Professor of Experienced Based Education at Sinclair College, Ohio, USA, and Dr Thembisile Khanyile, a Senior Lecturer, School of Nursing and Midwifery, University of Natal, Kwa Zulu Natal, South Africa.
- Chapter 3 draws upon emergent benchmarks for APL practice in order to identify a common set of guidelines and procedures for the assessment of prior learning.
- Chapter 4 presents case studies of APL practice within colleges, universities and the professions. Examples of developmental, credit exchange and *complementary* approaches are given, including examples from the USA, the UK and Canada. The chapter concludes by drawing together emergent themes and trends, which are applicable to APL practice.
- Chapter 5 examines in more detail a *complementary* approach towards APL, and the techniques used for portfolio development and appraisal.
- Chapter 6 promotes the use of a study guide, so you can plan appropriate developmental activities to maintain and continuously improve your APL practice.

## HOW TO USE THIS BOOK

- You can, if you wish, participate in a series of *key learning activities*. These will enable you to reflect upon, and continuously improve, your practice of assessment of prior learning. Feedback on these key learning activities is given on page 103.
- A *glossary* of terms is provided on page 101.
- A *reading list* is provided on page 96.

# 1 ASSESSMENT OF PRIOR LEARNING (APL): THE UK EXPERIENCE

This chapter will describe the concept of APL and its theoretical underpinnings. It will discuss the potential benefit of APL to learners, employers and education institutions. It will also describe the relationship of APL to the establishment of a credit-based system, and the factors which might influence the development of this. Finally, this chapter will identify emerging benchmarks for practice, and how these are being used to resolve issues which are currently influencing the APL process.

At the end of this chapter, you will be able to:

- describe what is meant by *assessment of prior learning* (APL)
- identify the benefits of APL for learners, employers and education institutions
- outline the educational principles which underpin APL practice
- identify factors which are currently influencing APL policy and practice
- identify guidelines and benchmarks for APL practice.

## WHAT IS ASSESSMENT OF PRIOR LEARNING?

Assessment of prior learning (APL) is the general term used for the award of academic credit on the basis of learning that has occurred at some time in the past. This learning may have come about as the result of a programme of study, or as the result of experience gained at work or during voluntary activities, in the home or during leisure pursuits.

The credit that may be awarded by an education institution, on the basis of prior learning, may take the form of access or entry into a programme of study. It may take the form of exemption or advanced standing within a course of study. It might also involve certification or part credit towards an academic award.

The type and amount of credit that is awarded is based on certificates the learner has gained which demonstrate that learning has already been assessed, or it may take into account learning from experience. Credit is awarded for learning that can be demonstrated, not for the experience itself. This credit is considered to be of equal standing to that awarded to others who have followed a traditional course or programme of study.

APL is of particular value to adult learners wishing to return to formal education, or to reduce the overall time spent on a programme or course of study. Adult learners wishing to seek credit via APL can do so on the basis of learning acquired at work, through voluntary work or from leisure activities.

They may also do this on the basis of non-certificated learning from self-directed study, certificated learning from other educational institutions, and certificated work-based learning.

Although APL can be used as a means of access or entry into educational institutions, the ways in which prior learning is now being used by learners is becoming increasingly varied. For example, prior learning may be assessed and used for access to a programme of education and training, for exemption from modules or units within programmes of education and training, or the award of a qualification or credential.

Within the UK, APL has particularly been developed within the context of competence-based education, for example, in the UK National Vocational Qualifications or NVQs. The assessment of existing competence, regardless of how or where this competence was achieved, is a fundamental principle of NVQ philosophy. The same principle is also fundamental to the practice of the assessment of prior learning. Also, within UK further education colleges and universities, APL appears to have developed as an integral part of articulation agreements, or credit and accumulation and transfer (CATs) schemes.

## APL AND ADULT LEARNING

APL originally started in the USA, in the 1970s, as a research project entitled 'The Co-operative Assessment of Experiential Learning'. From this project, in 1974, the Council for Adult and Experiential Learning (CAEL) was formed under the leadership of Dr Morris Keeton who indicates that:

> *CAEL was founded on two rather simple commonsense ideas: that what a learner knows and can do should be recognized appropriately no matter how or where it was learned and that hands-on experience of things being learned about and worked with can enhance that learning.*

> Keeton (2000: 47)

Keeton's views are consistent with those expressed by early adult learning theorists, such as Carl Rogers (1969) and Malcolm Knowles (1980), see below.

---

### The beliefs of two early adult learning theorists

**Carl Rogers (1969)**
- All human beings have a natural potential to learn.
- Significant learning occurs when the learner perceives the relevance of the subject matter.
- Learning involves a change in self-organization and self-perception.
- Learning that threatens self-perception is more easily perceived and assimilated when external threats are at a minimum.

---

- Learning occurs when the self is not threatened.
- Much significant learning is acquired by doing.
- Learning is facilitated when the learner participates responsibly in the learning process.
- Independence, creativity and self-reliance are all facilitated when self-criticism, and self-evaluation is integrated into the learning process.
- Much social useful learning is learning the process of learning and retaining an openness to experience, so that the process of change may be incorporated into the self.

### Malcolm Knowles (1980)
- The adult learner is self-directive.
- For the adult learner, experience becomes an exceedingly rich resource in learning.
- Adults learn from the problems with which they are confronted, and which they regard as relevant.
- Adult learners are more problem-centred than subject-centred.

More recently Kasworm and Marienau (1997) have established five principles of adult-orientated assessment practice:

- It recognizes multiple sources of knowing.
- It recognizes and reinforces the cognitive, conative and affective domains of learning.
- It focuses on adults' active involvement in learning and assessment processes, including self-assessment.
- It embraces adult learners' involvement in and impact on the broader world of work, family and community.
- It accommodates adults learners' increasing differentiation from one another, given varied life experiences and education.

## APL: DEFINITION, TERMINOLOGY AND SCOPE

Assessment of prior learning (APL) is defined as a systematic process that involves the identification, documentation, assessment and recognition of learning (i.e. skills, knowledge and values). This learning may be acquired through formal and informal study including work and life experience, training, independent study, volunteer work, travel, and hobbies and family experiences.

Assessment of prior learning (APL) can be used toward the requirements of education and training programmes, occupational and/or professional certification, labour market entry, and organizational and human resource capacity building.

Challis (1993) states that the goals of APL include:

- the identification of learning, wherever it has taken place

- the selection of that learning which is relevant to a desired outcome, career or occupation
- demonstration of the validity and appropriateness of the learning
- matching learning outcomes to those stated within a chosen accreditation framework
- assessment of evidence against criteria to ensure the validity of the claimed learning
- accreditation within an appropriate and recognized accreditation framework.

One of the difficulties encountered in trying to understand APL is the range of acronyms that are often used by different people, and in different countries. For example, in the United States, APL is known as *prior learning assessment* or PLA; in Canada, it is known as *prior learning assessment and recognition* or PLAR; in South Africa and Australia, it is known as *recognition of prior learning* or RPL.

In the UK, the term AP(E)L is generally used as an all-encompassing term to include prior certificated learning, as well as prior experiential learning. Within the UK, AP(E)L includes:

- *accreditation of prior achievements* (APA), for example, National Vocational Qualifications (NVQs) where the claimant exchanges proof of past achievements in the workplace for unit credits within a nationally-agreed vocational framework
- *accreditation of prior certificated learning* (APCL) – learning for which certification has been awarded by an educational institution or another education or training provider
- *accreditation of prior experiential learning* (APEL) – non-certificated learning gained from experience. APEL is sometimes referred to as RPEL (*recognition of prior experiential learning*).

## THE BENEFITS OF APL

As well as an instrument for accreditation or recognition, APL can also be used as a diagnostic tool for identifying training needs, for example, to assist companies to determine the competence of their workforce, prior to planning future training and development activities. APL can also be used as an initial assessment process to allow individuals with non-standard entry qualifications to gain access to university programmes. Finally, APL can be used as a free-standing assessment facility to enable students to earn credit for their prior learning and to have this formally recognized by the award of credit towards a qualification.

A University and Colleges Advisory Service (UCAS) survey of practice, carried out in the UK in 1996, indicates that APL is used in a wide range of programmes, at both undergraduate and postgraduate levels, particularly in nursing, social work and management programmes. In their study, UCAS (1996) indicate that APL has benefits for wide and diverse groups of learners, many of whom may not have had the opportunity to participate in university education before. This may include unemployed people seeking recognition for past work experience, either for access, or advanced standing, also people with certificated or non-certificated work-based learning seeking credit for a university award, those seeking to 'top up' an existing qualification, for example, certificate plus work experience towards a diploma or degree. It may also be beneficial for people who have left a course of study before completion, who now wish that learning to count towards another award. The benefits of APL for learners, employers/managers and university staff are outlined below.

---

### The benefits of APL

For learners:
- Credit achieved through APL can be used to access programmes leading to particular qualifications.
- Credit achieved can be counted as part of the total credit required for particular awards, and may shorten the time taken to gain a qualification.
- Recognition of learning from experience, and the process of reflection required to construct a claim often leads to an increased level of confidence.
- Preparing a claim for APL helps to develop independent study skills.
- Reflection on experiential learning enhances the link between theory and practice.

For employers/managers:
- APL may lead to an accelerated path to a qualification, and thus less time spent away from the workplace.
- APL is less costly than fees for taught modules.
- The process of reflection on practice may lead to innovation within the workplace.

For university staff:
- APL encourages curriculum innovation as new techniques for assessment are developed.
- The process encourages study to be relevant to work, life and personal development.
- Claims are made on the basis of recent experience – this often provides rich material for discussion and can stimulate research partnerships with employers.

adapted from UCAS (1996)

---

Merrifield *et al.* (2000: 50) state that APL has the following benefits for students, universities and employers.

- For students:

  *APL is both a validation and a learning tool. It recognizes and values what they know. It also develops lifelong learning skills: managing their own learning, identifying strengths and needs, developing confidence and self-awareness through reflection.*

- For employers:

  *APL offers the chance to increase the qualifications of their employees while minimizing time lost from work. By its focus on applied learning or learning in action, APEL helps individuals make learning transfers.*

  Merrifield *et al.* (2000: 4)

- For universities:

  *APL attracts mature, experienced learners to higher education. It can support partnerships with employers and community organizations. It provides tools to assess learning wherever it happens, can be a catalyst for innovative teaching and learning practices, and relates to academic and learning support staff through the Institute for Learning and Teaching.*

  Merrifield et al. (2000: 4)

## PRINCIPLES UNDERPINNING APL

Assessment of prior learning is a process of continuous assessment that may involve *formative* (diagnostic) as well as *summative* (terminal) assessment. It may include assessment of educational documents, portfolio review, demonstration or challenge processes (e.g. written/oral examinations, projects, assignments, performance observation, skill demonstrations, simulations and product assessments), standardized tests and programme review. In order to demonstrate rigor, the process must be *valid, reliable* and *sufficient*:

- *Validity* Assessment should be based upon the required outcomes or competencies, and their associated criteria. Assessment is said to be valid if the assessor refers only to the stated criteria.
- *Reliability* is concerned with the consistency of assessment – the degree to which an assessor's opinion may match that of another assessor in the same situation, with a similar adult learner using the same criteria.
- *Sufficiency* In order that an assessment may be deemed to be sufficient, adult learners must be able to demonstrate that all criteria within each of the specified outcomes have been met, including any necessary underpinning knowledge and understanding, where appropriate.

APL evidence must also be:

- *current* – up-to-date
- *authentic* – the individual's own work.

In order for a college or university to successfully offer APL, it must develop, or work within, a credit-based system which clearly defines:

- *credit* – a means of quantifying any learning that has been achieved
- *level indicators* of the demand, complexity and depth of study undertaken by the learner
- *level descriptors* – statements describing the expectations of each level of study
- *learning outcomes* – statements that describe what a learner should know, understand and/or be able to do
- *assessment criteria* – statements that are used to demonstrate that learning outcomes have been achieved
- *notional learning time* – the length of time that will be taken, on average, to achieve the learning outcomes
- *module or units of learning* – a self-contained 'block' of learning which makes up a course or programme of study.

SEEC (undated)

A good example can be found within the UK, where the above principles have been applied to a national system for delivery of National Vocational Qualifications (NVQs).

## NVQs: A NATIONAL CREDIT-BASED SYSTEM

In the UK, the Qualifications and Curriculum Authority (QCA) endorses NVQs. These are qualifications based upon the skills, knowledge and understanding required for competence within a particular occupational area. NVQs are concerned with outcomes rather than the learning process and individuals may gain an NVQ in a variety of ways: through a formal training programme leading to an award, through a mixture of formal, informal or open learning approaches, or through their past experience. NVQs allow open access to all, regardless of age, sex, race, special needs or prior qualifications. Individuals are given an opportunity to progress through a nationally-recognized framework of qualifications based upon achieving competence no matter how it is acquired.

In order that a National Vocational Qualification can be endorsed by QCA it must be based upon national standards required for performance in employment. The award must also be free from any barriers which restrict access and progression and available to all those who are able to reach the required standard by whatever means.

All NVQs are accredited within a nationally-agreed credit framework according to progressive levels of achievement and areas of competence. Refinements to the framework are made as qualifications are developed and routes for progression and transfer are identified. The function of the framework is to provide a coherent classification for NVQs and to facilitate transfer and progression both within areas of competence and between them. The areas of competence defined in the framework are derived from an analysis of work roles, and provide the organizing structure for all competence-based qualifications within England, Wales and Northern Ireland. In Scotland these qualifications are known as Scottish Vocational Qualifications (SVQs).

Currently the national framework defines eleven areas of occupational competence, for example construction, engineering and manufacturing. NVQs are being developed to cover areas of competence at all *levels*, from the application of basic skills to professional understanding (see below).

---

### Level indicators within the NVQ framework

**Level 1:** Competence in a range of routine and predictable work activities

**Level 2:** Competence in a variety of work activities, some complex and non-routine, ability to work both alone and in collaboration with others in different situations

**Level 3:** Competence in a variety of mainly complex and non-routine work activities in differing situations, often while controlling or guiding others

**Level 4:** Competence in a wide range of complex, technical or professional work activities in differing situations, often with responsibility for both other staff and allocation of resources

**Level 5:** Competence involving the application of fundamental principles and complex techniques in a wide and often unpredictable range of work situations, together with responsibility for other people's work and the allocation of substantial resources

NCVQ (1989: 10)

---

At each level within the national framework, an NVQ is made up of several *units of competence*. A unit is defined as the smallest grouping of performance standards that makes up a key task or function within an occupational area. Each unit of competence is made up of several *elements* (descriptions of employment expectations) and their associated *performance criteria* (the critical performances required in the workplace). (See Figure 1.1.)

The responsibility for occupational standards development rests with employers and trades unions. These are determined using the process of discussion, consultation and research. The principle method of standards development uses the process of functional analysis. This involves experts from an occupational area identifying the key purpose of that occupation by observing individuals going about their daily work. Subsequent analysis of these observations results in the generation of a statement about what the employee has to do, and any qualifying factor. Thus a statement of key purpose could be written as follows:

DO  / SOMETHING / TO AN AGREED STANDARD
(Verb) /   (Object)   /            (Condition)          McCrory (1992: 25)

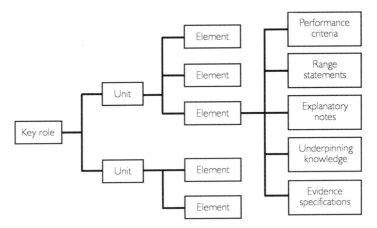

**Figure 1.1**    NVQs, units, elements and performance criteria (Care Sector Consortium, 1992: iii)

Each statement of key purpose (a unit) is further divided into elements (a description of key activities that make up a unit), each element being further divided into the standards of performance required in order to successfully complete a key occupational role (performance criteria) – see Figure 1.1.

Elements of competence also have *range statements* linked to them, these specify the breadth or area of work which a candidate is expected to display within an occupational area. Explanatory notes are sometimes attached to the range statements to provide further explanation of required performance.

Finally, *underpinning knowledge* and *evidence specifications* detail the type and amount of evidence or information which needs to be gathered in order to safely infer a person's competence during assessment and to highlight the knowledge and skills that a candidate should be able to demonstrate across the range. An example of an NVQ unit within the care sector, showing unit title, unit elements and performance criteria is given below.

---

### NVQ units, elements and performance criteria: an example from the care sector

Unit 0: Promote equality for all individuals

**Elements of Unit 0**
0.a    Promote anti-discriminatory practice
0.b    Maintain the confidentiality of information
0.c    Promote and support individual rights and choice within service delivery
0.d    Acknowledge individuals' personal beliefs and identity
0.e    Support individuals through effective communication

---

**Performance criteria for Element 0.a**

0.a.1   anti-discriminatory practice is promoted in ways which are consistent with the worker's role and legislation and charters concerning individual rights

0.a.2   the worker's behaviour in the work setting demonstrates recognized good anti-discriminatory practice and is not exploitative or abusive

0.a.3   where the worker is unsure of appropriate forms of behaviour for specific individuals or has discriminatory feelings towards an individual, the appropriate advice, guidance and support is sought.

0.a.4   where an individual directs discriminatory behaviour to the worker, the appropriate action is taken to the behaviour or support is sought

0.a.5   where an individual makes inappropriate or discriminatory actions or remarks, the effects or consequences of her/his actions are explained in a manner, and at a level and pace, appropriate to her/him

0.a.6   where an individual is at risk from abuse, exploitation and discrimination by others, the appropriate action is taken to support the individual

0.a.7   discriminatory behaviour from others is responded to in an appropriate manner and consistent with agreements made with the work team

0.a.8   where an individual wishes to make a complaint about discriminatory practice, s/he is appropriately supported in doing so

adapted from Care Sector Consortium (1992)

## FACTORS INFLUENCING APL PRACTICE

Within the last decade, the UK government has challenged education institutions to widen access to further and higher education, and to increase throughput of students, at no extra cost to the taxpayer. As a result of this dynamic, interest in APL has increased. However, unlike other pedagogical approaches, the practice of APL has not been developed or refined through a process of systematic and rigorous enquiry (Trowler, 1996). Rather, it has been based upon 'happenstance, coincidences and flukes of timing' (Evans, 2000: 49). This has led to much scepticism, as well as resistance towards the practice of APL within colleges and universities (see below).

### Attitudes towards APL

**Enthusiasts,** whose commitment to the introduction of credit systems is driven by a crusade for access, democratic participation and institutional reform, but some of whom may be unaware of alternative ideological positions in play;

**Pragmatists,** for whom the introduction of credit systems seems to offer plausible solutions to sectoral and environmental changes, and who may or may not be informed by particular ideologies or educational objectives;

**Sceptics,** who are open to persuasion on the need for changes, question the appropriateness of many proposals, doubt the permanence of changes, and many of whom remain evenly balanced between their support for educational change and their desire to retain familiar academic practice;

**Antagonists,** who largely reject the entire enterprise for a number of different reasons, ranging from expressions of vested interest through to expressions of deep-seated intellectual disquiet.

adapted from HEQC (1994: 314)

Perhaps its not surprising, therefore, that APL has been subject to much controversy. For example, there is ongoing debate concerning the relative value of learning gained outside the formal education system. This debate serves to reinforce existing tensions between employers, students and education providers, and creates barriers for individuals wishing to have their non-formal learning recognized and accredited. This phenomena is often referred to as *academic gate-keeping*. It is an indicator of the power relationship which exists between the learner and faculty member, and can influence the APL process (Trowler, 1996).

 **Key learning activity I**

Using the guidelines outlined in Chapter 6, obtain the following article: Trowler, P. (1996) Angels in marble? Accrediting prior experiential learning in higher education, *Studies in Higher Education,* Vol. 21, No. 1, pp 17–30.

Using the guidelines for critical reading in Chapter 6, summarize possible biases in the APL process – you might want to organize these under the headings of *Cultural, Educational* or *Organizational.*

Do you feel these biases are any different to those found within traditional forms of assessment?

In addition to the cultural, educational and organizational issues identified by Trowler (1996), there have also been some concerns regarding the clarity and transparency of the APL process. For example, Paczuska and Randall (1996) state:

> ... *procedures are frequently informal, may be poorly documented, and implicit in admissions practice and in any credit awarded, rather than explicit. For the prospective student the process may be inaccessible unless they happen to come into contact with a particular individual tutor. For*

*tutors and guidance workers who advise prospective students the details are
so often unclear.*

Also, in a recent UK study, Merrifield *et al.* (2000: 3) indicate that although APL
practice has been developing since the 1980s, it is still an area which is not well
known or understood by students or academics. In particular, Merrifield *et al.*
indicate that mechanisms for APL are unwieldy and are not user-friendly, nor
are the potential benefits of APL well known to employers. The authors
conclude that a gap between policy and practice exists.

Similar concerns regarding APL practice have been acknowledged by SEEC
(1995: 15), who, when launching a quality code of practice, state:

> *The need to provide a Code of Practice for AP(E)L has come from a growing
> recognition that a set of established common principles have underpinned the
> operation of AP(E)L and that these should be made more explicit than they
> have generally been.*

However, despite SEEC's early attempt to introduce a code of practice, recent
studies conclude that comprehensive information concerning APL and its procedures is still generally unavailable. What is available is often misunderstood. As a
consequence, Merrifield *et al.* (2000) recommend that:

> *higher education institutions must make information about the potential for
> AP(E)L widely accessible.*

They further recommend that higher education institutions should:

> *review each element of their own practice against a variety of good practices
> that have been developed in different contexts.*

This issue is also taken up by the UK Quality Assurance Agency for Higher
Education (QAA, 2000: 6) who state that in designing and operating assessment
processes, higher education institutions should consider:

> *how to make information and guidance on assessment clear, accurate and
> consistent and accessible to all staff, students, placement or practice assessors
> and external examiners.*

QAA further state that such information should include 'any role played by
Accreditation of Prior (Experiential) Learning and the processes involved' (QAA,
2000: 17).

## GUIDELINES AND STANDARDS FOR PRACTICE

In an attempt to standardize the APL process, emphasis has recently been placed
upon the establishment of guidelines, firstly in the USA, by the Council for Adult
and Experiential Learning (CAEL). These state the following:

- Credit should be awarded only for learning and not for experience.

- College credit should be awarded only for college-level learning.
- Credit should be awarded only for learning that has a balance, appropriate to the subject, between theory and practical application.
- The determination of competence levels and of credit awards must be made by appropriate subject-matter and academic experts.
- Credit should be appropriate to the academic context in which it is accepted.
- Credit awards and their transcript entries should be monitored to avoid giving credit twice for the same learning.
- Policies and procedures applied to assessment, including provision for appeal, should be fully disclosed and prominently available.
- Fees charged for assessment should be based on the services performed in the process and not determined by the amount of credit awarded.
- All personnel involved in the assessment of learning should receive adequate training for the functions they perform, and there should be provision for their continued professional development.
- Assessment programmes should be regularly monitored, reviewed, evaluated, and revised as needed to reflect changes in the needs being served and in the state of the assessment arts.

Established in 1989, the CAEL guidelines primarily address organizational issues for APL. However the importance of these guidelines cannot be overstated, for they have significantly influenced both policy and practice internationally.

## Canada

In 1997, the Canadian Labour Force Development Board (CLFDB) published the following minimum standards for PLAR:

- PLAR must be accessible and relevant to people as individuals. It must focus on the unique needs and abilities of the individual.
- Assessment and recognition must be of learning (knowledge and skills acquired through study or experience) not of experience.
- The PLAR process must be fair and equitable. It must be barrier-free and bias-free.
- The PLAR process must be efficient. It must make the best use of resources for the individual.
- The PLAR process must be effective. It must provide the opportunity for recognition of prior learning, but it must not hold out false promise.
- The PLAR process must be transparent. The individual must know the criteria and standards used to assess his or her skills and knowledge.
- The assessment must be reliable. The criteria and standards must be recognized and respected by all the labour market partners. This principle applies to occupational and skills standards, the learning outcomes stated for a specific course or training programme, and the credentials required for a specific job or occupational group.
- The assessment tools and their PLAR application must be recognized and accepted by all the labour market partners.

- Individuals assessing prior learning must be trained to perform this task.
- The assessing organization must provide a number of ways to carry out an assessment.
- Individuals should have the opportunity to choose how their assessment will be done. If necessary, they should get help to make their choice.
- Recognition awarded through PLAR should be considered equal to recognition awarded in the traditional manner.
- Recognition awarded through PLAR should be transferable between organizations, provinces and territories.
- PLAR must be an option or opportunity, not a mandatory process.
- If a person is not satisfied with the PLAR assessment, an appeal procedure must be available.

The influence of CAEL is apparent within these guidelines, but the CLFDB only address organizational issues, with no real attempt to define or illuminate the role of the practitioner, the learner or the APL process.

## United Kingdom

In an attempt to clarify the role of the APL practitioner and the learner, the UK South East Education Consortium (SEEC) published their code of practice for APL in 1995. This included the following operational guidelines:

- Information about AP(E)L should be accessible to all applicants.
- Where academic staff are involved in the guidance and counselling of students in the preparation of AP(E)L evidence, they should not normally be the sole assessors of that evidence.
- The role and responsibilities of students will be made explicit in the AP(E)L process.
- Experience on its own is insufficient grounds for gaining credit. APEL credits the learning which the learner can evidence from prior experience.
- Evidence of learning must be assessed by academic staff using whatever means are appropriate.
- The AP(E)L process must be equitable and capable of scrutiny and enhance quality.
- Charges for AP(E)L, where they occur, and the criteria for these, should be clear to students and the institution.
- Where there is a maximum and/or minimum volume of credit allowed for AP(E)L, such limits should be made clear.

Despite SEEC's attempt to introduce some clarity into the process, five years later a study by Merrifield *et al.* (2000) concluded that comprehensive information concerning APL and its procedures was still generally unavailable within UK universities.

**Key learning activity 2**

Obtain a copy of your own organization's guidelines for APL practice, and compare these with the CAEL, CLFDB or SEEC guidelines.

What similarities or differences do you notice?

Discuss with your APL co-ordinator, or a respected colleague, how these similarities or differences might influence the role of the APL practitioner?

---

OCCUPATIONAL STANDARDS FOR APL PRACTITIONERS

## United Kingdom

In order to clarify the process of APL, recent emphasis has been placed upon the development of standards for practitioners. A good example in the UK is the work of the Training and Development Lead Body (1995), who have identified the competencies required of the APL adviser, through the process of *functional analysis*.

The TDLB standards outline the key purpose, functions, activities and performance indicators relating to the work of assessors. A key purpose is a functional definition of an occupational group, e.g. *all* assessors including APL assessors. It identifies why things are done (a *function*) not what things are done (a *task*). A function describes how the key purpose is to be achieved. An activity indicates how the key function is to be achieved. *Performance indicators* indicate the standard to be achieved within the field of APL.

According to the TDLB, the key purpose of an assessor is to:

> *review progress and to assess achievement, so that individuals and organizations can achieve their education and training objectives.*

According to the TDLB the functions and activities of assessors are to:

- *prepare the candidate for assessment.* This includes the following activities:
  - help the candidate to identify relevant learning
  - agree to and review an action plan for demonstration of prior learning
  - help the candidate to prepare and present evidence for assessment
- *assess the candidate.* This includes the following activities:
  - agree to and review an assessment
  - judge evidence and provide feedback
  - make an assessment decision using differing sources of evidence and provide feedback.

The use of this approach in universities is highly controversial and is anathema to many academics, as it represents a mechanistic or behavioural view of learning, which (it is claimed) introduces the potential for both social and political control (Day, 1996).

## DEVELOPING BENCHMARKS FOR APL

## Canada

In order to clarify the process of APL, the Canadian Association for Prior Learning Assessment (CAPLA) have adapted the work of the TDLB (1995) and devised benchmarks for APL practice (see: http://www.tyendinaga.net/fnti/prior/benchmarks.htm).

Benchmarks for APL can be beneficial, for example, CAPLA conclude that benchmarking is:

> *a process that tends to build consensus and can be used in combination with other methods of job analysis.*

Day (2000: 124)

and also confirm that:

> *the process of benchmarking has a high degree of internal validity and it is sensitive to the qualities, characteristics and processes that help to define Practitioner behaviour.*

Day (2000: 124)

Benchmarking is a continuous, systematic search for, and implementation of, best practices that may lead to improved performance. The goals of benchmarking are to build on the success of others, and to address current best practice. Benchmarking for APL is a beneficial process as it:

- *focuses on client needs* – this is fundamental to adult learning
- *adapts industry-best practices* – best practice from education institutions
- *helps to set relevant, realistic and achievable goals* – an open and transparent process for individuals and assessors
- *tests the quality of programme delivery* – students, employers and educational institutions must be able to see that the process is rigorous and credible.

The strengths, weaknesses, opportunities and potential threats of using benchmarks for APL are outlined below.

---

### *Strengths, weaknesses, opportunities and threats of benchmarks for APL*

**Strengths**
- Use of benchmarks will ensure that APL will become a defensible process.
- Provides a sense of reliability, equality and fairness.
- Improves accountability and transparency in the assessment process.
- Identifies what is possible, what is feasible, and what is acceptable.
- Ensures consistency of approach, particularly for workplace-based assessment.
- Will improve the rigor and fairness of the assessment process.

---

- Identifies the resources needed for assessment.
- Individuals will become more aware of requirements for assessment, thereby improving access to APL.
- Protects the rights of the learner.
- There will be more direction for faculty, thereby increasing confidence in the process.
- Provides a common understanding and communication between stakeholders.
- Identifies an ethical process for the professional.
- Improves mobility for the assessor.

## Weaknesses
- Potential cultural or class bias.
- The language and standard adopted may be inappropriate.
- Danger of a 'cookie cutter approach', i.e. one size fits all.
- There is a potential conflict of interest if a practitioner advises and assesses.
- Costly – will only happen if government funding is available or if employers can commit the resources.

## Opportunities
- There is little information on APL available – practitioners will welcome the direction that benchmarks can provide.
- Can provide a methodology and/or a process for adult learning, e.g. learning in the workplace; the promotion of client-centred approaches to learning.
- Can assist in the accreditation and articulation process between institutions.
- Can be used as a basis for training and certification; this will lead to credibility and acceptance of the assessor role.
- Benchmarks for APL may be transferable, e.g. quality audit, workplace assessment, academic assessment.
- Can give credibility to what are traditionally known as 'soft' skills, e.g. employability skills, by identifying a rigorous and consistent approach for assessment.
- Can motivate educational institutions to define curricula in outcomes-based language.

## Potential threats
- The individual or the assessor may see benchmarks as unrealistic expectations.
- Benchmarks may redefine the role of the practitioner – a potential threat for faculty.
- Assessors will come under greater scrutiny, especially if there is an appeal.

- There may be a demand for 'perfection' by the purchasers and commissioners of education.
- Universities may reject any prescriptive process or 'top down' approaches to certification of practitioners, e.g. from government departments.
- Traditional values and beliefs about assessment may well generate resistance, e.g. a credential is only valuable if few people possess it.
- Potential bureaucracy of assessment, e.g. N/SVQs.
- Risk of reductionism, i.e. there may be a 'whole' which is overlooked.

adapted from Day (2000)

According to the CAPLA (Day, 2000; 2001), the key purpose of the APL assessor is to:

*review progress and/or assess achievements, so that individuals and organizations can achieve their personal development and/or education and training objectives.*

The performance indicators relating to each of the functions and activities of the APL practitioner are outlined in Appendix 1 and are examined in greater detail in Chapter 3.

## SUMMARY

This chapter has described the concept of APL and its relationship to adult learning theory. The principles which are fundamental to rigorous assessment of prior learning and the establishment of a credit-based system have also been discussed.

The potential benefits of APL to learners, employers and education institutions have been outlined and emerging guidelines and benchmarks for practice have been identified in an attempt to make the role of the APL practitioner much more explicit and transparent.

Finally, the cultural, social, organisational and educational factors which might influence APL practice have been highlighted. The next chapter re-examines these issues in the light of international developments in APL practice.

# 2 ASSESSMENT OF PRIOR LEARNING: INTERNATIONAL PERSPECTIVES

This chapter re-examines the cultural, social, organizational and educational factors which might influence APL practice. It does this within an international context by considering recent developments in prior learning assessment, both in the USA and South Africa.

In this chapter, the concept of *prior learning assessment* (PLA) and its determinants is discussed by Professor Carolyn Mann, Sinclair College, Ohio, USA, and the concept of *recognition of prior learning* (RPL) is discussed by Dr Thembisile Khanyile, School of Nursing and Midwifery, University of Natal, Kwa Zulu Natal, South Africa.

At the end of this chapter, you will have identified cultural, social, organizational and educational factors currently influencing international APL policy and practice.

## USA AND PRIOR LEARNING ASSESSMENT

### The context

The nature of modern American society has become more complex and interdependent; changes in competition, technology, information processing and lifestyles are all interacting to affect the way we lead our personal and professional lives. Continuous life-long learning is essential for the development of strong economies necessary to compete in a global marketplace. New partnerships and alliances between educational institutions and a host of organizations are blurring traditional educational boundaries. These forces have converged to place increased pressure on colleges and universities to face the reality of change and embrace new processes and approaches to teaching and learning (Rowely, Lyan and Dolence, 1998). Numerous leaders are calling for a paradigm shift in order to better serve the educational needs of the information age (Barr and Tagg, 1995; Maehl, 2000; O'Banion, 1997). Barr and Tagg (1995) argue that the traditional approaches of the *instructional paradigm* no longer accommodate the needs of today's world. O'Banion (1997) suggests that we are on the wave of a reform that places learning as the central value and activity of the educational enterprise. The instructional paradigm, which has long been the dominant paradigm, places emphasis on the delivery of instruction in a classroom setting by the faculty expert. Students are typically viewed as passive receptors of the faculty's knowledge. The new paradigm, often referred to as the *learning paradigm*, shifts the focus to learning acquired by the learner, and away from the delivery of instruction by academic experts; and what appears to be a subtle difference has immense impact on educational institutions. The type of competencies necessary for the information age and how students master the appropriate knowledge, skills and attitudes becomes the crucial focus for educational institutions, not where or who delivers the instruction. Placing more emphasis on learning and less importance on who delivers the learning will result in colleges and universities not being the only institutions involved in facilitating and supporting life-long learning. This shift requires a far more collaborative approach between educational institutions and learners. The key components of continuous life-long learning that community colleges must address are: open and flexible access; the growth of learning networks and partnerships; and the recognition of learning wherever it takes place (i.e. the assessment of prior learning).

## Historical developments

During the last thirty years, the award of college credit for prior learning has grown from an experimental project to a recognized programme for adult learners completing academic degrees (Gamson, 1989; Whitaker, 1994). The first formal system for assessing prior learning in the United States was the General Educational Development Examination (GED). This programme was designed during World War II under the oversight of the American Council on Education (ACE) to assess the educational growth of service men and women who had left high school to serve in the armed forces. After the war, ACE extended the programme, using the GED examinations to demonstrate high-school equivalency for the civilian population.

Throughout the 1940s, 1950s and 1960s the pressure on higher education to serve the adult student continued to build (Gamson, 1989). By the end of 1946, one million veterans had taken advantage of the GI Bill and by the end of the eligibility period in 1956 over two million veterans had used their benefits (Rose, 1989; 1990). The Department of Defence teamed up with the American Council on Education (ACE) in the early 1940s to take a serious look at the comparability of service training programmes with college learning. Before the end of the war, the Educational Testing Service (ETS) of Princeton, New Jersey, and ACE began evaluating military training and experience to determine civilian educational equivalency (American Council on Education, 2001).

By 1947 ACE and the Department of Defence undertook a more ambitious project to evaluate some of the military occupational specialties (MOS) and training conducted by the armed forces to determine their comparability to college and university courses (American Council on Education, 2001). Using college and university faculty and staff, ACE established guidelines, procedures and criteria for assessing both military training programmes and occupational specialties. Where equivalency existed, they recommended that colleges and universities consider awarding appropriate credit hours to the military personnel who had completed the trainings or attained the military occupational specialty (MOS) levels. ACE established guidelines for colleges and universities to use in awarding the credit and worked with GIs to petition for the credit at various colleges and universities.

The United States Armed Forces Institute (USAFI) developed a parallel project aimed at helping colleges and universities respond to adult students returning from the armed services. During the war, USAFI provided correspondence courses and other educational materials to soldiers. Once the war was over USAFI also began offering testing and accreditation services to parlay learning soldiers had acquired into currency recognizable, and creditable, by high schools and colleges.

Several early experiments with assessment of prior learning and accelerated degree programmes for adults on the collegiate front were conducted. In 1954 Brooklyn College was perhaps the first to award credits directly to adults on the basis of the assessment of previous experience (Gamson, 1989). The University of Oklahoma in 1957 designed one of the first baccalaureate programmes for adults. In 1963 Queens College, City University of New York (CUNY) began a special programme for adults: the Adult Collegiate Education Program, which gave formal recognition, in the form of college credit, to adult students for what they had learned through their life and work experiences In the following years Florida International University, Antioch College, Goddard College, and several other colleges, developed unique programmes for adult students for recognizing and crediting their prior experiential learning.

Assessment opportunities for adults began to become more prevalent in higher education during the late 1960s and early 1970s. According to the Continuing Education Association, the number of part-time adult learners enrolled in American colleges and universities almost tripled, growing from just under 2 million to almost 6 million (National University Continuing Education Association, 1990). A number of social shifts were contributing to the increase in adult students in higher education and the necessity of higher education to accommodate adults on their terms (Cross, 1994). These factors forced higher education to re-evaluate two questions: (1) who was it serving? and (2) how was it serving the learners? By the 1960s, the social, economic and educational pressures contributed not only to the increase in adult students but also to the necessity of higher education to accommodate adults on their terms (American Council on Education, 2001; Gamson, 1989).

While a variety of non-traditional programmes had been established by the early 1970s, the pivotal influence on the development of individualized prior learning recognition programmes evolved from the Commission on Non-Traditional Study. The Commission, established in 1971, was a joint undertaking of the Educational Testing Service (ETS) and the College Board. The Commission recommended that colleges and universities make themselves more accessible to adult and part-time students by creating alternative avenues by which students could earn degrees, as well as complete a major portion of their work for a degree (Gamson, 1989). The Commission emphasized the need to develop a variety of new ways to assess what students learned from life experiences. In 1974, based on the Commission's findings a small group of colleges and universities formed the Cooperative Assessment of Experiential Learning (CAEL) to develop and implement sound academic practices regarding the awarding of college credit for non-academic learning experiences, placing particular emphasis on the development of the portfolio process. Under the leadership of Morris Keeton and supported by funds from Educational Testing Services (ETS) and later the W.K. Kellogg Foundation, early CAEL associates have served the dual role of educators and change agents to promote and develop methods to assess prior learning (Gamson, 1989). Their work has been instrumental in the development and support of assessment of prior learning programmes at numerous colleges and universities (Tate, 1999).

## Definition, rationale and scope of prior learning assessment

Prior learning assessment is a process of evaluating and granting college credit for learning that has taken place outside of academic control, using such methods as examination, programme evaluation and individualized approaches. Prior learning is defined as the learning acquired from non-academic life or work experience that has occurred prior to formal contact with a college or university. Adults are often involved in a variety of learning activities that are not sponsored or directed by higher education. The types of learning activities are endless and the oversight of the activities is equally as varied. A great deal of learning is occurring in the workplace – the American Society for Training and Development (ASTD) estimated that business and industry spends $30 billion annually on training (Maehl, 2000). A great deal of learning is informal and structured by the learner. Tough's early study (1967) of adult learners found that 90 per cent of adults are involved in at least one learning activity annually. The average learner conducts five learning activities, investing an average of 100 hours per learning effort; the learner plans 80 per cent of all learning projects.

Two underlying arguments have contributed to the growth of assessment of prior learning programmes: the democratization of higher education and the growth of experiential learning. As the idea of a more democratic higher education system began to enter the public consciousness in the early 1970s, individuals and organizations began to question the *status quo* (Gamson, 1989). Possessing the appropriate credentials is essential in a highly mobile, technical society (Maehl, 2000). We live in a society not only where credentials are increasingly important, but also where the alternatives for people without credentials are becoming fewer. Access to the credentialing process is largely contingent on the amount of higher education one has completed. Possession of a degree enhances an individual's access to power and impacts on almost every phase of life, affecting confidence, competence, advancement and income. Colleges and universities have recognized policies and expanded programmes and services with the goal of making the academy more accessible to diverse groups of students.

Prior learning assessment has been viewed as a means of widening access to higher education for people whom by virtue of their age, gender, race, socio-economic background and/or prior educational qualifications have been denied entry. More recently, the application of the assessment of prior learning has expanded as a means to gaining entry to professions, to participate in training and development opportunities by employees and as a means to decide if individuals possess the skills and knowledge to advance in their jobs (Keeton, 1999). It is becoming increasingly associated with notions of economic regeneration and retraining, as well as the need for continuing education to cope with the technological changes and the needs of the knowledge explosion (Craft, Evans and Keeton, 1997; Gamson, 1989; Maehl, 2000).

The educative rationale for assessment of prior learning is grounded in the experiential learning theory's notion that knowledge is valid regardless of the source. Learning is the focus of assessment of prior learning not where the learning occurred. The academic recognition of prior learning shifts the focus of an institution to the learner and their learning and away from the focus on location or who is sponsoring the learning experience where the learning occurred or the notion of seat time.

Simply stated, experiential learning means learning by doing (Merriam and Caffarella, 1999); learning is grounded in the experience of the learner. This theory presents a fundamentally different view of the learning process from that of the behaviourist theories of learning. The theory provides a more holistic perspective on learning that combines experience, perception, cognition and behaviour. Learning is the process where concepts are derived from and continually modified by an individual's experience. The key elements of experiential learning are that learners analyse their experience, evaluate and reconstruct their experiences in order to extract meaning from it in the light of previous experiences. Ideas are not fixed but are formed and reformed from one's experiences.

Experiential educators feel that all experiences could be the source of learning, thus giving rise to the need to recognize and assess learning from life experiences for college credit. Experiential education has been viewed by many as a means of providing a framework for examining and strengthening the linkages between education, work and personal development (Kolb, 1984; Sheckley and Keeton, 1994).

Advocates of experiential learning theory argue that good educational practice demands a more holistic approach when serving adults than was historically applied to traditional-aged students. One of the fundamental characteristics that distinguish adult learners from traditional college students is the years of experience they bring to a learning situation. Many educators have considered this to be one of the most important distinctions between traditional and non-traditional students. Educators have moved away from behaviourists' notion of teachers as purveyors of knowledge and learners as passive receptors. Current cognitive, humanistic and constructivists learning models stress the importance of meaning formation (Merriam and Caffarella, 1999). Learning is viewed as an active process where an individual takes an idea, concept or problem and makes it their own by integrating the new learning into their own knowledge and experience (Barr and Tagg, 1995; Cross, 1994; O'Banion, 1997). Models of good practice in adult education are placing more emphasis on the utilization of learners' previous experience in order to enhance current and future learning. Recently there has been an increased recognition by adult higher educators that the need to make sense of one's life experiences and what one knows can serve as an incentive for adults to engage in learning activities (Lewis and Williams, 1994). The reflection and assessment of past experiences and prior knowledge has served as a motivator for adult learners to modify, transfer and reintegrate what those experiences mean in terms of their values and beliefs, as well as the knowledge, skills and abilities they possess (Clark, 1993; Daloz, 1986; Meizrow, 1991).

## Practice issues

How is assessment of prior learning practised in the United States? There are three basic approaches that are commonly used by educational institutions to award credit for prior learning. These are:

- tests
- evaluation of non-college sponsored training
- assessment of individualized portfolios.

### Testing

Testing is still the predominate method used by colleges and universities. Two categories of examinations are used to evaluate prior learning: external, standardized examinations and internal, proficiency/challenge examinations. Standardized tests have been developed and marketed by such groups as the Educational Testing Services (ETS) and the American College Testing (ACT) for a number of subject areas. A committee of experts prepares the examinations, and the test results are compared against traditional college courses to develop normative scores. Numerous academic institutions recognize credit for the achievement of a minimum score of these external exams. College and university faculty often prepare their own internal examinations courses as a means to evaluate prior learning. These internal examinations expand the range of subject areas available to students, and allows individual faculty to be more directly involved in both the preparation of the test and the evaluation of the individual learner.

### Evaluation of non-college sponsored training

As previously discussed, the American Council on Education (ACE) has evaluated military training and made college credit recommendations for colleges and universities to consider for awarding credit for learning. In 1974, ACE expanded this process to include the evaluations of ongoing training programmes for college credit to non-military organizations under the auspices of their College Credit Recommendation Services (ACE/CREDIT; note the programme was first called the Program on Non-Collegiate Sponsored Instruction, PONSI). Their recommendations are published in the National Guide to Educational Training Programs for colleges and universities to consider when awarding college credit. ACE/CREDIT evaluations, modelled after the military programme, are conducted by teams of subject-matter experts drawn from a variety of academic institutions. The variables used to determine college credit are the intended learning outcomes, the length of time, the levels of complexity and the methods employed to evaluate the participant's achievement of the learning outcomes.

Prior learning is not always easily categorized into a traditional subject area, thus standardized tests may not be available to assess a student's learning. Even when prior learning is easily related to a specific subject area, such as drafting or quality management, there may not be a standard examination available. In addition, the prospect of testing makes many adult learners very uncomfortable. And merely offering a test does not address the issues of how to help adult learners know what tests to take or how these tests relate to their career and academic goals. ACE/CREDIT recommendations are applicable for only those organizations that have contracted to have their training programmes reviewed. Neither of these method provides a mechanism to assist individuals with the process of evaluating their own learning or how to develop a plan to enhance or build upon previous knowledge.

**Portfolios**

The method most closely associated with the assessment of prior learning is the use of student-prepared portfolios as an evaluation tool. A recent CAEL survey found that 52 per cent of the colleges and universities surveyed use portfolios as a means for assessing prior learning (Zucker *et al.*, 1999). The portfolio process offers both methodological and educational advantages over the other two methods. Advising and assisting learners to identify college-level learning and how such learning relates to the students' overall degree plan are crucial components of a portfolio process. Through this process of assessing their learning from experience, students develop a working model of their own learning process, expand their understanding of how they construct their world view, improve their self-directed learning skills and apply all of this to the completion of their life-long learning goals (Sheckley and Keeton, 1994). Standardized tests, oral interviews, performance assessment and programme evaluations (ACE) are often incorporated into the portfolio process, allowing both individuals and faculty to take advantage of all three methods.

Most institutions provide a *portfolio development workshop* or credit course to assist students. In developing a portfolio, students are assessing their own learning with the assistance of a faculty member. Early definition of the portfolio focused on the physical document. A portfolio is the formal document that details learning acquired through non-college experiences used to request college recognition for the learning from experience. Typically, a portfolio includes the following: autobiographical information, goals statement, description of learning in the form of an essay or a three-column format typically referred to as a competency, and documentation to support the learning.

The definition of a portfolio expanded as practitioners placed more emphasis on reflection and the learning associated with the process itself. The word has come to represent the process of identifying, articulating and documenting non-college learning for academic purposes. The preparation of a portfolio is an exercise in self-evaluation, introspection, analysis and synthesis. It is an educational experience in itself. Students are guided through a process that requires them to relate their past learning experiences to their educational goals, to exhibit critical self-analysis, and to demonstrate their ability to organize documentation in a clear, concise manner.

Students develop a better understanding of how their learning relates to an academic degree. They identify their strengths and weaknesses, and how the curriculum can help address their weaknesses and capitalize on their strengths. Preparing a prior learning portfolio is not an easy task. Thus, a student should not be asked or expected to do so without careful consideration of the educational value of the process, and how the process directly relates to the student's achievement of academic goals. The development of a portfolio and its subsequent evaluation should be part of the individual's educational programme. The goal of the process should be to enhance the value of education for the individual.

College and universities that have developed strong assessment of prior learning programmes have focused on three essential obligations in assessing and crediting prior experiential learning:

> *to develop a sensible rationale for the experiential learning that is consistent with the institution's mission, reasonable in relation to its resources, and useful to its intended clientele;*

> *to translate that rationale into workable policies, guidelines, and operating procedures that are made clearly known to all students and interested parties; and*

> *to insure that these policies, guidelines, and procedures are followed with reasonable fairness and consistency and useful outcome.*

> Willingham (1977: 5)

Whitaker's '10 standards for quality assurance in assessing learning for credit' (Whitaker, 1989) have come to be viewed as the essential tenets of assessment of prior learning. The principles are divided into two categories: the academic standards and the administrative standards. On the academic side, the good-practice principles focus on assessment process of identifying, articulating, documenting, measuring, evaluating and transcribing learning; on the administration side, the standards focus on policy and procedure, guidelines, assessors, costs and quality control.

## Sinclair Community College

Sinclair Community College (SCC) is a comprehensive community college offering over 2,000 different credit courses with over 80 associate and certificate degree programmes. Currently, 21,000 full- and part-time students attend SCC with an additional 40,000 individuals involved in training activities through the Division of Corporate and Community Services. SCC has a long history of serving the needs of adult learners since its beginning in 1887 as a YMCA college offering evening courses. Currently, the average age of students is 32 years and 53 per cent of the student population is 25 years or older.

The real emphasis on the assessment of prior learning began in the mid-1970s with the development of the Credit for Lifelong Learning Program (CLLP). The college recognized college credit for standardized examinations (i.e. College Level Examination Program and Advanced Placement Program) and internal proficiency examinations as early as 1972. Under the leadership of Dr Barry Heermann, the momentum to implement assessment of prior learning as an educational programme was spurred by the following factors:

- faculty's interest in serving the needs of their adult students
- recognition that learning is a life-long process
- the growth of learning activities taking place outside of direct college sponsorship.

Under the auspices of the Experience Based Education Department (EBE), the college has developed a comprehensive programme using a variety of methods, examinations, programme evaluations and portfolio assessment to assist students with the recognition of college-level learning from prior learning experiences. Sinclair faculty members have awarded over 56,000 credit hours of college credit, with 22,000 hours being awarded from the evaluation of 7,000 portfolios by 203 faculty evaluators. The strength of Sinclair's assessment of prior learning programme is grounded in four factors:

- the involvement of academic faculty in the award on academic credit
- the number of assessment options available
- the integration of assessment of prior learning into the academic institution
- the college's commitment to expanding access to all learners.

The college placed a great deal of effort on developing faculty support for the concept of assessing prior learning, actively involving faculty from all divisions in early discussions and implementation decisions. While the EBE department oversees the assessment of prior learning, SCC faculty determine the award of credit and have the autonomy to determine assessment methods. Prior learning, and not prior experience, was firmly established as the basis for credit award.

Sinclair's Prior Learning Portfolio Development course has served as an anchor for the Credit for Lifelong Learning Program since the programme's inception. The basic objectives of the three-credit-hour course are to:

- help adults identify their learning from experience
- match their learning to college-level courses
- develop a portfolio which articulates and documents their request for Sinclair courses.

Sinclair's programme is a course-match process, meaning that, with the assistance of a portfolio faculty, students identify specific courses for which they prepare a portfolio, articulating and documenting how their learning from experience matches the course competencies.

At Sinclair, a portfolio prepared by a student contains the following components:

- *a cover letter*, which states the student's credit request
- a 4–5 page *life history*, which outlines significant events and how these events affected the student
- a 1–2 page *goals paper*, which describes the student's personal, career and educational goals
- a year-by-year *chronological record*, listing experiences since graduating from high school
- a *narrative of learning*, describing how the student learned the material covered
- *documentation* of learning experiences to support the competency course
- a concise discussion of the course objectives – this is also referred to as a *competency*.

The competency is the heart of the portfolio; using a specific three-column format, the student outlines the experiences that have been significant in his or her learning about the objectives for a specific course and discusses what he or she has learned about the course objectives. Documentation is provided to verify and support the student's credit request. Once a portfolio is submitted to the faculty for evaluation, the faculty member reads the document and has the option to interview the student. The faculty evaluator can ask the student to provide additional work or participate in other types of assessment techniques that they deem necessary to help them decide if the student should receive credit and what grade should be recorded.

With the help of a portfolio faculty resource person and other Experience Based Education staff members, a student progresses through the following steps in the portfolio development process:

1 Proving adequate, college-level reading and writing skills, the student enrols in the Portfolio Development class, in a section offered at a convenient time and place.
2 Through a series of exercises, the student reflects on his or her life and prepares a chronological record and life history paper.
3 The student clarifies his or her educational, career and personal goals in the light of past growth/experiences, and develops a short goals paper.
4 With the assistance of the portfolio faculty resource person (and consultation with an academic counsellor, if needed), the student identifies and records the college-level learning he or she has acquired through non-classroom sources, relating it to classes offered at Sinclair, to demonstrate equivalency.
5 The student documents the college-level learning claimed.

6  The student completes the portfolio, which includes a statement of educational, career and personal objectives, a chronological record, a clarification of experiences and related learning, and supportive documentation. The portfolio shows how the learning cited is related to particular courses or competencies. The student's request for credit hours commensurate with his or her learning is also included.

7  The portfolio is reviewed by Credit for Lifelong Learning resource faculty persons, and returned to the student with their comments, for revisions or corrections as warranted.

8  The student pays for individual evaluations of all competencies developed.

9  Individual teaching faculty evaluates the portfolio.

10  The student is awarded credit commensurate with demonstrated learning.

## Evaluating the impact of prior learning assessment

The most basic question regarding assessment of prior learning is asked by both faculty and students: Is it worth it? Institutions have found that creating an assessment of prior learning programme has assisted faculty to improve their classroom teaching because they must clearly articulate their expectations. Students are attracted to institutions with prior learning programmes, and they stay to complete their degrees at those institutions. Business and industry are attracted to institutions with assessment of prior learning programmes because they view such programmes as a benefit for their employees and as a means to encourage employees to pursue academic degrees. The initial contact has created partnerships in other areas between the two groups to the benefit of both.

Is it worth the effort for the student? When presented with the alternative of taking a class that is a repetition of prior learning, thousands of students have chosen prior learning assessment. In addition to the academic recognition, the process helps students set realistic goals and develop educational plans. Students understand their level of expertise and how it relates to their degree plans. Students' self-esteem increases as they receive validation of their learning experiences from prior experiences. The evaluation of assessment of prior learning is important, but it must be done in the context of helping individuals achieve academic and career goals. Otherwise, why go to the trouble of identifying, articulating and documenting learning if there is no path to continue after this process?

Faculty cannot assume that students will continue to pursue academic goals in the traditional manner after assessment of prior learning. Successful assessment of prior learning programmes have numerous non-traditional options to complete degree requirements. Assessment of prior learning is designed around the broader context of empowering adult learners. Learners need a variety of non-traditional ways to continue to meet their career and academic goals.

Prior learning assessment requires that faculty be actively involved in the process and committed to assisting the learner. Faculty must examine their philosophy of learning and often refocus on their primary customer, the learner. In order for assessment of prior learning to be successful, faculty assumptions about teaching and learning must be challenged in a way to help faculty move towards a learning paradigm. Assessment of prior learning, particularly the use of portfolios, has always been a controversial issue in higher education. The basic tenets challenge the traditional views of the instructional paradigm, challenging many faculty and administrators' assumptions about the teaching and learning process. College-level learning within this paradigm could only take place in a college classroom under the auspices of a trained faculty member. Faculty, who once controlled the entire learning process, are asked to shift perspectives to the role of evaluators of learning in which they had no direct involvement.

Procedures must be developed to guide students through the entire process; faculty input is essential for each step. Faculty must develop criterion standards, detailing what they mean by college-level learning to assist students as they prepare portfolios, as well as guide the evaluation of the portfolios.

Finally, commitment is required of the student. Developing a portfolio is a complex task, requiring students to review their experiences, extract the learning and articulate that learning form that faculty can evaluate for college credit. Students must become actively involved in the learning process. Faculty must assist and support the student's commitment.

## SOUTH AFRICA AND RECOGNITION OF PRIOR LEARNING

The need to transform the education system in South Africa has been a subject of intense debate and discussions since the early 1970s. The systemic investigation undertaken by the Committee of University Principals (CUP) in 1987 brought important issues to the fore, thereby emphasizing the importance of quality and uniform standards in South Africa. This investigation revealed that standards varied from a level which can be compared with the best international universities, to standards that were barely acceptable at tertiary level (CUP, 1987: 100). The reason for these disparities was the legacy of the apartheid system of government which led to inequality of the education standards among educational institutions.

With the inception of the democratically elected government in 1994, the Department of Education was challenged with the responsibility to bring about justice and equality in education. This coupled with other related changes from the economical and technological environment in South Africa, necessitated action. After 1994, the then education minister committed his department to the concept of a single co-ordinated system of education and training. This system would ensure that access to higher education is expanded within the context of limited increase in public expenditure. The concept implied a rethinking of the entire education system, as well as a transformation of curricula and programmes. To be successfully implemented, this concept of a single education system for the country called for the development of new policies with new sets of goals and mechanisms to realize those goals. Emphasis was put on mechanisms that would enhance quality while affording equality. Quality was important for this new system if it was to be comparable at international levels. Equality was also important if the system was to be sensitive to past imbalances in education and training caused by the previous system of education in the country. It was these challenges that led to the development of a new quality assurance system within the broad ambit of the South African Qualifications Authority (National Commission on Higher Education Report, 1997: 247). Subsequently, the National Qualifications Framework (NQF) was established. According to the NQF, higher education programmes would be registered within a single coherent qualifications framework, based on a laddered set of qualifications from higher education certificates and diplomas to masters and doctoral degrees. For the first time in South Africa, the stakeholders of education and training, namely the government, business sector education and training providers, and community organizations, were all represented in the generation, registration and reviewing of standards.

## The NQF and recognition of prior learning

The recognition of prior learning (RPL) is one of the most exciting, yet challenging and contested, cornerstones of the National Qualifications Framework. It is exciting because it holds the potential for the recognition of knowledge, skills and competencies of people who had been denied learning opportunities within the formal education sector, and who have therefore been overlooked as competent in their places of work precisely because of their lack of formal certification. RPL is challenging because it is a difficult and complex process that is inextricably bound into prevailing social relations of power and knowledge. It is contested because these social relations reflect different, and sometimes conflicting, views and approaches to education and training between different social partners such as education and training, organized labour, business and communities. For instance, while the labour sector approach and understand RPL from a socio-political perspective, the education and training sector views it as a challenge to the only power they have, the power to name what counts as knowledge and how that knowledge should be demonstrated. It is these conflicting views about RPL that have triggered a broad public debate about the concept.

## A framework for implementation of RPL

Since 1994 the government has made rapid progress in building the new foundations for a co-ordinated national system of education and training, with the provision for national and provincial competencies. The first seven years have seen the government focus its work on the development of the South African Qualifications Authority (SAQA) and the NQF, and on the Employment Equity Strategy and the Skills Development Strategy. Each of these frameworks will now be discussed briefly to highlight their influence on the implementation of the RPL principle.

The National Qualifications Framework aims at facilitating access to, and mobility and progression within, education, training and career paths. The NQF is also aimed at accelerating the redress of past unfair discrimination in education, training and employment opportunities and thereby contributes to full personal development of each learner and the social and economic development of the nation at large. As mentioned earlier, RPL is the major principle of the NQF. According to SAQA, affirmative action should ensure equal opportunities on all levels for historically disadvantaged citizens. SAQA describes a 'qualification' as that obtained from formal learning, prior learning and relevant experience, as well as the ability to acquire competency in a reasonable time. SAQA challenges business to recognize informal and non-certificated learning. It also challenges education and training providers to consider other forms of learning, and not only learning which takes place within the classroom. The NQF has as its major aim the improvement of the vocational skills of employees in such a way that these skills are registerable with SAQA, and are in line with the National Qualifications Framework.

The Skills Development Act has also made provisions for the establishment of the Sector Education and Training Authorities (SETAs) to develop and implement sector appropriate education and training plans that will meet the economic and social development agendas. Education and Training Quality Assurance bodies (ETQAs) will be established by the SETAs to accredit and monitor the quality of education and training provision within their sectors. Therefore, the providers of education and training together with their ETQAs are required by the SAQA to implement RPL so as to ensure that the country's goal of education for social development is achieved.

## Different approaches to RPL implementation

According to Dewey, as cited in Tanner and Tanner (1980), one cannot penetrate deeply into any significant educational problems or issues without encountering philosophical considerations (Tanner and Tanner, 1980: 102). This is also true of RPL as its philosophical basis can shed clarity on how the meaning of the concept is understood. This is an important consideration in South Africa given the number of stakeholders involved in the generation and monitoring of educational standards. As a consequence three different and contrasting views of RPL have emerged:

- the technical approach
- the progressive approach
- the radical approach.

### The technical approach

All education is consumer-oriented and utilitarian. Education is viewed mainly in terms of its usefulness to the labour market. Knowledge is a means to the economic end and is value-free. Knowledge is viewed in normative terms as a product, which is visible and therefore potentially measurable. The purpose of RPL in this approach would be to provide a baseline for planning in order to achieve a particular target, for example 100 per cent competence of the workforce. The focus here is on competence and hence the assessors are not interested in the individual's new learning or development. This approach has been mostly influential in the RPL projects initiated by the business sector (COSATU, 2000: 67).

### The progressive approach

Education is an instrument of social and political reform. Education is aimed at bringing about the development of a whole person within the society with that which is useful to the individual as the main focus. Knowledge in this approach is inseparable from experience. Human beings are regarded as the creators of knowledge, therefore RPL in this approach is seen as a challenge to the academic standards with its fast tracking systems of credits. Academics using this approach only view RPL as a means of opening up access for more adult learners to re-enter the education system. For them, RPL practices should be distant from the main stream. As long as these adult learners can produce enough evidence that their previous experience 'fits in' with the existing learning outcomes for the particular programmes, then they will be accepted. Previous experience has to be manipulated to conform to the canonical boundaries of knowledge. There is no attempt for the providers of RPL in making the educational programmes flexible enough to accommodate adult learners and their previous experience. This approach has found a comfortable place in most higher education institutions.

### The radical approach

Education is not neutral, therefore it can only be understood by locating it within its historical contexts. Education should seek to explore that which is oppressive and dominating. The focus being on bringing about a new social order. Knowledge in this approach is obtained through a dialogue and engagement within the society, therefore the context is the source of knowledge. As learners interrogate their own learning experiences, they are able to give them new meaning. In other words, they begin to see their previous experiences in a new light. This leads to growth and development of the whole society. The purpose of RPL in this approach is social transformation of the whole society through the transformation of the educational system. In this way, the very curricula and standards can be informed and even changed by RPL practices.

## The different contexts of RPL

According to Harris (2000), formal work on RPL began in 1994 when the National Training Board (NTB) established a sub-committee of an existing working group to address assessment issues. The introduction of a single co-ordinated education and training system with an aim of redressing past imbalances in education positioned the RPL as the key principle of the National Qualifications Framework that had a capacity for such issues of redress. RPL experiences in the country have been broadly located within the *workplace* and in *higher education*.

## RPL in the workplace

RPL in the workplace in South Africa dates back to the early 1990s when representatives of organized labour sought the recognition of workplace-based and experiential learning for the purpose of job grading and access to further education and training for their members. A number of pilot projects were implemented in the mining, auto and construction industries, but these were far less successful in meeting the different purposes of employers, unions and the workers than was originally hoped. Very few workers succeeded in gaining the recognition they sought. The reasons given for the failure of these projects according to Ralph (2001) were:

- The assessment methods and standards used were those imported from other countries like Australia and these did not match the South African-based experiences of those who were assessed.
- The standards were written by experts who used academic-based language which an ordinary person in the workplace was not familiar with.
- These projects were dominated by management since the workers were not represented in the planning stages of the project.
- The very purpose of RPL was viewed by workers as threatening since the project's main objective was to assess productivity of the workforce. In other words, the RPL purpose was a skills audit. The workers felt threatened by the inevitability of retrenchments.
- The assessors themselves lacked adequate training in the whole RPL process.

As a response to these problems, in 2000 the Council for South African Trade Unions (COSATU) took an initiative to counter what they viewed as inherent contradictions of human capital approach to education, training and assessment. COSATU embarked on a broad research project to analyse the RPL activities in the workplace. The result of this project was a publication of a manual which served as a guide to unions involved with RPL implementation in the workplace. The main objective of the manual was to ensure that RPL processes, if implemented, do not act against the country's main objective of RPL which is social transformation (Vavi, 2000). It would appear, therefore, that the business sector was influenced by the technical approach.

## RPL in higher education

Universities, although historically underpinned by the liberal human progressivist tradition in which experience is valued, have traditionally not valued experience either in terms of accreditation or as a measure within teaching and support. Experience is seen as a means towards the academic end (Harris, 1997). As the boundaries for higher education continue to weaken, knowledge is less strongly classified and framed, and the market rather than social class becomes the deciding factor (Bernstein 1996: 101). The challenge, therefore, is that RPL is the key principle of the National Qualifications Framework (NQF) and is to be followed across all sectors.

Some institutions, like the University of Cape Town, the University of the

Orange Free State, the University of Natal, the Peninsula Technikon and the University of Port Elizabeth, have already started pilot programmes with RPL. For example, in 1996, the University of the Free State, in partnership with De Paul University, the Joint Education Trust and the Council for Adult Experiential Learning, embarked on a project to start a bridging programme for adult learners in management positions who did not have the necessary qualification. The outcome of this project saw the commencement of a portfolio development course which served as a bridging programme for those without matriculation but who wished to be admitted into a university degree. This was the first experientially-based management and leadership degree and was offered through the faculty of Economics and Management Sciences. Learner support mechanisms included an in-house library and contact sessions during weekends. Methods of delivery included problem-solving, dialogue and presentations. Assessment strategies included oral examinations and assignments (Anderson, 1998).

The University of Natal School of Nursing has been involved in a major RPL project for nurses in South Africa since 1998. The project's main objective was the development of a model for RPL for South African nurses. Once developed, the model was pilot-tested in three nursing education institutions in Kwa Zulu Natal: Natal College of Nursing with all its four campuses; Prince Mshiyeni School of Nursing and the School of Nursing's Decentralized Programmes at the University of Natal. In the Free State province, it was the Free State School of Nursing with all its three campuses.

A developmental approach to RPL implementation emerged where adult learners were supported through portfolio development to submit evidence of prior learning and also to fill in deficits in their prior knowledge. This approach helped the learners to incorporate old and new learning. All institutions involved used different methods of assessment like portfolios, practical examinations and theory examination. The success of this project was attributed to the collaborative nature of stakeholder involvement. The outcome of this project was that all institutions involved have continued implementing RPL for adult learners. The University of Natal School of Nursing has since commenced with a course for RPL facilitation aimed at helping those educators wishing to gain skill in the whole process of RPL. A separate portfolio development course has also commenced at this institution for adult learners wishing to access programmes of nursing (Khanyile, 2000)

The South African Nursing Council as the Education and Training Quality Assurance body for nurses in 2000 took the initiative and developed a policy for RPL implementation in the country. The Council formulated guidelines based on the South African Qualification Authority and these were refined by the stakeholders. Nursing education institutions are expected to use these guidelines as basis for their own institutional policies on RPL (Khanyile, 2000: 102).

## A unique approach to RPL

There are three main factors which make the South African approach towards RPL unique:

- *RPL is a government policy.* Recognition of prior learning policies in South Africa has been placed at the centre of the attempt to put down the unspeakable inequalities of the past and create a democratic civil society. In countries like the UK and New Zealand, RPL practices have evolved largely within vocational and academic contexts. In South Africa, the government through the Ministry of Education is the key role-player, driving the transformation of the education and training system. Whilst in other countries RPL has been an activity of individual institutions, in South Africa it is a government policy. All education and training institutions are required by the government to implement this policy.
- *The purpose of RPL is social transformation.* According to the National Plan for Higher Education, the main objectives for all these new policies is equity, quality and social development. In South Africa, RPL is a major social imperative, in other words RPL implementation should ensure social transformation.
- *The South African RPL candidate may be different.* The South African situation is somewhat different since RPL candidates might have their experiential learning constructed under very disadvantaged conditions. These candidates may have a wealth of experience but could have very low levels of formal education, having the instruction medium as a second language and being drawn from largely working-class communities with no socialisation to academic discourse. On this basis, the situation is a complex one since a balance between recognising prior learning and rectifying past inequalities will make recognition of prior learning difficult to fit easily into the traditional higher education categories (Usher and Edwards, 1995: 123).

Therefore a successful model for RPL implementation will be one that takes into consideration the above mentioned factors. In particular, a more developmental or holistic model is advocated, which during assessment will take into consideration both old and new learning, as well as the context under which this learning was obtained.

Experiences of implementing RPL within South Africa have revealed the importance of *social context*. Importing RPL models from one country into another without any consideration for indigenous cultural, social and political issues may be problematic. Collaboration between all stakeholders during RPL implementation is also important, since many will share differing perspectives about the purpose, or even the meaning of the concept.

In South Africa, RPL is fundamental to social transformation, to the restructuring of many social institutions, from workplace to universities. Recognition of prior learning holds potential for restitution and social redress both in education institutions, and in the workplace. For academics, RPL provides the challenge to redefine sources of knowledge, sites of knowledge acquisition and the nature of knowledge. These factors, coupled with a traditional view that academic standards and assessment cannot be explicitly articulated, have combined to make RPL a difficult concept to implement within an academic context (McMillan, 1997: 45).

## SUMMARY

This chapter has examined factors influencing the policy and practice of APL. It has done this within an international context by considering recent developments in the USA and South Africa. You are now invited to compare developments in these two countries with APL practice in the UK and, in particular, to identify any similarities or differences in the approach. This will help you to contextualize the cultural, social, organizational and educational factors currently influencing APL policy and practice. The following key learning activity will assist you to do this.

 **Key learning activity 3**

Look back on Chapters 1 and 2 and answer the following questions.

1 What are the principles of 'adult orientated' assessment?
2 How do these principles relate to APL?
3 How would you define assessment of prior learning?
4 Does your own organization have an acronym for assessment of prior learning?
5 Summarize the benefits of APL for the adult learner.
6 What are the fundamentals of a credit-based system?
7 What are the potential biases which might influence the APL process?
8 How do these differ from more traditional forms of assessment?
9 What are the principles underpinning rigorous assessment?
10 What are the main functions of the APL practitioner?

Don't forget to keep a record of your answers, as you may want to refer to these as you undertake other learning activities within this book.

You might want to use your answers as evidence towards a future claim for credit.

# 3 The role of the APL practitioner

The previous chapters described the concept of APL and its theoretical under-pinnings. They also outlined the potential benefits of APL, and the cultural, social and organizational factors currently influencing practice within South Africa, the UK and the USA.

In addition, Chapter 1 discussed how emerging guidelines and benchmarks are being used to resolve issues currently influencing APL practice. This chapter examines in more detail the role of the APL practitioner, drawing upon newly emerging benchmarks for practice in order to clarify the role of the APL adviser and assessor (Appendix 1).

At the end of this chapter, you will be able to:

- outline the *key purpose*, *functions* and *activities* of the APL practitioner
- outline the functions and activities of the *APL adviser*, *APL assessor* and *APL co-ordinator*
- identify key factors which might influence the role of the APL practitioner
- compare and contrast *direct* versus *indirect* evidence of prior learning.

## Definitions

An APL practitioner is an individual who utilizes learner-focused activities to formatively or summatively assess[1] an individual's prior learning either for academic credit or recognition of occupational and/or professional competence. The key purpose of an APL practitioner is to:

> *review progress and/or assess achievements, so that individuals and organizations can achieve their personal development and/or education and training objectives.*

> Day (2000)

This definition includes the work of the *APL adviser* who guides, assists and formatively assesses the learner – sometimes one-on-one, sometimes in small groups – in order to identify learning strengths and learning needs. It also

---

1 Formative assessment: 'designed to provide learners with feedback on progress and informs development, but does not contribute towards the overall assessment.' (QAA, 2000: 4).

　　Summative assessment: 'a measure of achievement or failure made in respect of a learner's performance in relation to the intended learning outcomes of the programme of study.' (QAA, 2000: 4).

includes the work of the *APL assessor* who summatively assesses individuals in order to award a final grade or to make a final decision about their competence.

APL assessors who summatively assess individuals should be competent and knowledgeable in the outcomes or competencies they are assessing. Within post-secondary education institutions, the assessor is usually a subject-matter expert from faculty. In workplace education and training programmes, the assessor is usually an experienced member of staff who is occupationally or professionally competent and is trained in assessment skills.

 **Key learning activity 4**

Review the Introduction to this book.

I How are you (or will you) be involved in the APL process? Are you (or will you) mainly undertake *formative* or *summative* assessments?

2 What potential biases or conflicts can you identify in your role as an APL practitioner?

Don't forget to record your answers. You might like to use a learning diary in order to do this (see Appendix 2).

An *APL co-ordinator* may be involved in the guidance and assessment of individuals, but will also be involved in maintaining, submitting and revising the use of assessment documents and records, for example, registration, orientation plans, assessment plans, assessment and certification procedures, appeals procedures; also, providing advice and support to advisers and assessors, for example, initial training, trouble-shooting, methods and resource development, continuing professional development and updating of assessors. The co-ordinator may also be involved in monitoring assessments and ensuring consistency in the assessment process, for example, establishment of sampling frameworks for the purpose of statistical analysis and report-writing, conducting regular assessor meetings for the purpose of developing consistency in assessment processes, individual needs and equal opportunities monitoring.

ESTABLISHING THE APL PRACTITIONER ROLE

When establishing their role, APL practitioners should expect to encounter some initial tensions within their organizations. Such tensions may arise in the following situations:

- between work colleagues who might question the rationale for selecting one person as a adviser or assessor, rather than another
- between APL assessor and manager, when the assessor negotiates time and space out of normal work activities in order to undertake assessments

- within individual APL assessors, particularly when they realize that they will be held accountable for their assessment decisions
- when individuals realize the need to reconcile the demands of being an APL assessor with the demands of being an APL adviser, so that objectivity can be maintained and any potential conflict of interest between the two roles can be avoided or minimized.

The APL practitioner's role demands a range of interactions with individuals from within and outside the organization. Interactions with adult learners include pre-assessment guidance and action planning, observation and ongoing collaboration and providing feedback on performance and/or competence. In addition, APL practitioners may be required to meet with their peers for the purpose of developing consistency in the application of assessment methods, meet with others in order to justify their assessment decisions (for example, APL advisers, APL co-ordinators, heads of faculty, heads of human resource development, external advisers, etc.) and liaise with adult learners, managers, administrators and faculty to report on individual progress and to comment on resources for APL.

It is essential that regular contact is maintained with faculty, other APL advisers and assessors, as well as with the APL co-ordinator so that competence in assessment and the integrity of the process is maintained. In order to competently carry out their duties, practitioners need to have a clear understanding of the process and how it relates to their role. They also need to have an appreciation of the competencies required of the adviser and the assessor (Appendix 1).

 **Key learning activity 5**

Review your responses to key learning activity 4 on page 39.

1   Did you identify any actual or potential conflicts or biases relating to your role as an APL practitioner? If so, how might these be resolved?
2   Draw up an action plan to assist you in developing your practitioner role. Indicate the factors which might be critical to your success and discuss these with your co-ordinator or a respected colleague.

Don't forget to record your answers. You could use the learning diary in Appendix 2 to do this.

At some point in their development, APL practitioners may need to demonstrate that they are competent in the relevant activities and functions outlined in Appendix 1. For example, what are the specific competencies which support the work of the APL adviser? These competencies are slightly different to those required of the assessor. The difference depends upon whether one is involved in formative or summative assessment. For example, the APL assessor will often make a final appraisal of an individual's work in order that academic credit can be awarded or competence confirmed, whereas the APL adviser is more often involved in informal or ongoing developmental work. The APL assessor carries out the following activities:

- agreeing to and reviewing an assessment plan
- judging evidence and providing feedback
- making an assessment decision and giving feedback.

Whereas the APL adviser mainly carries out the following activities:

- helping the individual to identify relevant learning
- agreeing to and reviewing an action plan for demonstration of prior learning
- helping the individual to prepare and present evidence for assessment.

Some activities are performed by both the adviser and the assessor. For example, both of these practitioners are involved in action planning, making an appropriate judgement about evidence and providing feedback to adult learners.

 **Key learning activity 6**

Compare your current (or intended role) as a practitioner with the functions and activities outlined in Appendix 1.

1  Would you say that you are (or will be) an APL adviser, an APL assessor, or both?
2  What activities (if any) differentiate the role of adviser and assessor within your organization?
3  Within your organization, what activities do the adviser and assessor have in common?

Record your answers in your learning diary (Appendix 2).

Many APL practitioners now undertake both roles as part of a team-based approach to assessment. Many assessment skills are common to both the adviser and the assessor roles. Each of the activities relating to the role of the assessor and the adviser are now outlined.

THE ROLE OF THE APL ASSESSOR

### Agreeing to and reviewing an assessment plan

Assessors may be involved in planning the most appropriate time, place and method for an individual's assessment. There is no prescribed format for this but they will need to take into account and discuss:

- the outcome or competence to be assessed
- an appropriate time and place for the assessment
- the type of evidence that needs to be gathered, e.g. how will competence be assessed as well as supporting knowledge and understanding?
- any aspects of confidentiality that may apply
- any ethical implications for assessment, e.g. how will the safety of a third party be maintained?
- any special assessment requirements – the individual may be a shift worker, nervous or use English or French as a second language
- the assessor and the adult learner need to make sure that they agree with the plan and that this agreement is appropriately recorded.

An example of an assessment plan is given in Figure 3.1.

## Judging evidence and providing feedback

APL practitioners may be involved in formatively or summatively reviewing the performance and/or competence of individuals, and evaluating them against the criteria for the competencies or outcomes being assessed. These outcomes or competencies should be made available to both the practitioner and the adult learner before an assessment is made of the learner's competence.

Practitioners are often required to review tasks and activities associated with the adult learner's field of study, place of work or chosen profession. This may be difficult to substantiate without the use of checklists or assessment records, which should be signed by the practitioner and the adult learner. To help validate an assessment decision, it is often useful to refer to examples of products that have arisen from the learner's work/studies. These products should be relevant to the criteria being assessed.

Practitioners will often need to ask questions in order to explore the supporting knowledge and understanding relating to the criteria which is being assessed. It is important not to lead the individual, i.e. that the question does not suggest the answer.

- Questions could be *spontaneous* – verbal questions arising naturally from the evidence being reviewed. It is advisable to jot them down, along with the adult learner's response, as far as is reasonably possible, i.e. do not let this distract from the work at hand.
- Questions could be *pre-planned* – a series of written questions necessary to ask of the individual, which are prepared in advance. APL practitioners and their colleagues could develop a question bank. This has the advantage that other assessors have checked the questions to ensure they directly relate to the criteria being assessed. These questions are confidential and should not be disclosed to individuals prior to the assessment.
- Questions could be *spontaneous and pre-planned* – as you become more familiar with the required criteria and more experienced in the art of interviewing, it may be possible to combine both strategies in order to get a greater appreciation of the individual's performance/competence and

Learner:   *Fred Smith*   **Adult learner identification no.** *00001*
**Organization:** *Peabody International*   **APL adviser/assessor:** *Malcolm Day*

**Outcomes/Competencies:**   **Criteria:** *Unit One H&S 1a, 1b, 1c*
*Peabody's Workplace Development Programme*
*Health and Safety at Work, Unit One*

**1. Assessment opportunities:**
*Fred is the workplace health and safety officer with responsibility for attending workplace accidents and administering first aid. He is also responsible for training other workers in first aid procedure. Evidence of Fred's competence can be provided by letters of validation from those whom he has assisted, plus records of incidents he has maintained (with client's permission). Fred always evaluates his training sessions; these evaluations are available in written form.*

**2. Assessment methods:**
Letter of validation: *3 validation letters from clients Fred has assisted.*
Workplace product: *copies of Fred's incident reports relating to the above.*
Workplace product: *copy of evaluation forms from at least 3 training sessions Fred has conducted.*
Interview/oral questioning: *Discuss the contents of Fred's portfolio and how these relate to criteria Unit One.*

**3. Resources required:**
*Blank letter of validation x 3*
*Copy portfolio development guidelines*

**4. Action to be taken by assessor/adviser:**
*Malcolm to provide Fred with blank copies of letter of validation, plus portfolio guidelines.*
*Malcolm to arrange interview to discuss Fred's portfolio and how it relates to criteria 1a, 1b, 1c.*

**5. Action to be taken by the learner:**
*Fred to compile a portfolio to include letters of validation, copy of incident records and copies of evaluation forms from training sessions.*
*Fred to get written permission from clients/administrators to use incident records.*
*Fred to let Malcolm have diary dates for meeting re: discussion of portfolio.*

Signature of adviser/assessor: _____   Date: _____

Signature of learner: _____   Date: _____

**Figure 3.1** An example assessment plan (adapted from Day, 1996, and Day and Zakos, 1999)

underpinning knowledge and understanding. Questions should cover processes, as well as outcomes. It is important to pay particular attention to situations which have not been verified by others.

Individuals can become extremely nervous when subjected to questioning. Questions are best kept simple and should be directly related to the criteria being assessed. A quiet room is needed, free from interruptions and distractions. Also, it is helpful to have a list of relevant questions on a separate sheet of paper to which to refer. The sheet of paper should also have a blank column in which to record the individual's answers. It is important to sign and date it and to get the adult learner's signature as well.

### Asking questions

When asking questions it is important to remember that learners have to first hear what is being said, then understand the question, think about it, search their memory, formulate an answer, then give the answer – this takes time. Remember to:

- ask questions in an interested manner and with a natural tone of voice
- word questions in simple and straightforward language – avoid textbook jargon
- pace the conversation and allow some time before going to the next question
- ask questions which require more than a yes/no response
- ask questions which only directly relate to the criteria being assessed
- pose questions which do not suggest the answer
- encourage the learner to give a full and complete answer.

Try to avoid:

- ambiguous questions
- trick questions
- repeating the learner's answer
- sarcasm at the wrong answers
- asking mainly factual questions
- repeating the question – it's probably better to rephrase it
- asking questions just to prolong the assessment
- asking questions that the learner will not be able to answer
- putting unnecessary pressure on the learner.

## Making an assessment decision and giving feedback

Once the evidence has been collected, the practitioner has to decide whether the individual has met the required criteria and inform him or her of the decision. Similarly if competencies or outcomes have not been met, the individual needs to be informed, in a positive and constructive way, how this gap can be filled. It is important to be clear and concise about this – in fact it is helpful to record this information for the person.

When giving personal feedback to the adult learner, it is important to be as

**Key learning activity 7**

Think back to an assessment you recently undertook with an adult learner.

1   How might you have improved your questioning technique?
2   Take one specific question that you used and indicate how you might have improved it.
3   Discuss your proposed improvement with a respected colleague. What does he or she think of your ideas?

Record your answers in your learning diary (Appendix 2).

---

sensitive as possible. Any negative comments may be harmful. It is also important to give the individual your undivided attention and to respond appropriately to how he or she may be feeling after the assessment. The discussion can be initiated by asking how the individual thought the assessment went – this will help to open up the feedback process and encourage him or her to share any concerns without fear of criticism. Individuals often identify gaps that have become obvious during the assessment process enabling the practitioner to build upon their strengths and work toward the development of a realistic plan to help overcome any shortfalls. It will take time to carry this out effectively. A quiet room, free from interruptions should help. However, it is your personal approach, the way in which interest and concern are expressed, that will help to ensure a successful outcome to this process.

### The interview

Interviews are an essential ingredient in the process. They provide both the adult learner and the assessor with an excellent opportunity to seek additional information, ask for clarification and engage in dialogue aimed at building on the learner's strengths and exploring realistic alternatives if additional learning/ evidence is needed. Skilled interviewers pay close attention to both verbal and non-verbal cues during the interview and respond appropriately to them.

During the interview, it is important to pay particular attention to the following factors which can have a significant impact on the outcomes of the interview:

- posture – relaxed, upright, facing the person at a reasonable distance
- gestures – balanced, open, relaxed and non-threatening
- facial expression – firm and pleasant
- eye contact – gentle, direct, relaxed gaze, same eye level
- voice, tone and volume – low-pitched, medium volume, gentle
- language – honest, open and to the point, giving praise and honest feedback, sharing and taking responsibility for your own feelings
- timing – putting your own point of view across and encouraging the learner to do the same.

Remember to record clearly and accurately the agreed-upon outcomes of the interview, identifying how any shortfalls can be overcome, the support the learner will need to overcome them and any agreed timelines. An example of an assessment record is given in Figure 3.2.

---

**Learner:** *Fred Smith*          **Adult learner identification no.** *00001*
**Organization:** *Peabody International*   **APL adviser/assessor:** *Malcolm Day*

**Outcomes/Competencies:**          **Criteria:** *Unit One H& S 1a, 1b,1c*
*Peabody's Workplace Development Programme*
*Health and Safety at Work, Unit One*

**Evidence methods used:**
*Discussion regarding Fred's role as a certified workplace health and safety officer, against criteria for H&S 1a, 1b and 1c (see portfolio) including administrative tasks and training role. A copy of the questions I asked are attached.*
*Three different letters of validation from those whom Fred has assisted (see portfolio) e.g. a client who fainted, a client who cut her hand and a client who suffered a heart attack.*
*Copies of evaluation sheets from 3 different training sessions Fred has conducted e.g. Principles of First Aid, CPR and fractures and sprains.*

**Areas where competence/outcomes have been achieved:**
*Fred has demonstrated that he is competent in all of the activities outlined in H&S Unit 1a, 1b, 1c.*

**Areas where competence/outcomes have not yet been achieved:**
*Fred is now collecting evidence relating to the Advanced First Aid at Work Module.*

**Assessor's comments (continue on back of sheet if you wish).**
*Responses to my questions (attached) and comprehensive workplace documentation placed in Fred's portfolio indicates that he is more than competent in the criteria required. Well done Fred!*

**Learner's comments (continue on back of sheet if you wish).**
*I was given very clear guidelines on to how to collect evidence against the criteria required. This made the compilation of the portfolio much easier.*

Signature of adviser/assessor: _____ Date: _____

Signature of learner: _____ Date: _____

---

**Figure 3.2**  A sample assessment record (adapted from Day, 1996, and Day and Zakos, 1999)

**Key learning activity 8**

Think back to an interview you recently undertook to give feedback to an adult learner.

1    How might you have improved your interview technique?
2    Take one particular aspect of the interview and indicate how you might have improved on it.
3    Discuss your proposed improvement with a respected colleague. What does he or she think of your ideas?

Use the learning diary in Appendix 2 to record your thoughts and ideas.

THE ROLE OF THE APL ADVISER

## Helping the individual to identify relevant learning

The APL adviser works with individuals and groups to help them identify relevant prior learning. It is possible to collect many forms of evidence to demonstrate prior learning. This section will concentrate on what is meant by *sufficient evidence* in relation to the use of a:

- learning diary
- letter of validation
- simulation.

### Learning diary

A learning diary can provide evidence that learners have the necessary supporting knowledge and understanding relating to an outcome or competence. When completed, the learning diary can be submitted to the assessor, who will then ask questions about it, for example, whether it is the learner's own work, how it relates to the criteria being assessed, as well as questions about the content of the material.

In keeping a learning diary, the learner will need to identify a strategy that will demonstrate that he or she has the appropriate knowledge relating to the criteria being assessed. For example, he or she may need to search out new and relevant information, read it, appraise it and record it in a meaningful way. The learner may also want to have a discussion with a more experienced colleague or mentor, or wish to attend a professional development activity or study day.

The learner will also need identify what he or she has learned, taking into account any reading, professional development activities and/or any discussions with others; then apply what he or she has learned to his or her practice by indicating how any new knowledge will be used in the workplace to solve a problem or deal with a contingency.

Finally the learner will identify the evidence he or she can use to demonstrate appropriate knowledge. This will need to be discussed with the assessor and it may include a bibliography, any notes taken, copies of any diagrams produced, any certificates received, etc. An example of a learning diary and how it might be completed is provided in Figure 3.3. A blank version is also provided in Appendix 2 for photocopying.

### Letter of validation

Validation letters can provide an indirect and authenticated account of the adult learner's performance/competence. They may be collected from colleagues, supervisors, managers, customers, suppliers, etc. Letters of validation should:

- be specific to an activity or product
- give a brief description of the circumstances and context of the observation
- give a brief description of the background and qualifications of the signatory
- give a brief background to the observed activity
- identify aspects of the outcome or competence demonstrated and how it relates to the set criteria.

It is helpful to provide a checklist for the individual writing the validation letter (the signatory) to link the learner's performance/competence directly to the appropriate outcome or competency.

The signatory may simply authenticate a piece of work as having been produced by the learner. In other cases, the signatory may provide an account of the learner's performance and comment on it in relation to the appropriate outcome or competency. It is important that signatories are familiar with the set criteria and are able to comment authoritatively on the learner's performance/ competence. Before accepting evidence from a letter of validation, the adviser will need to:

- judge the authenticity and validity of the evidence
- check that the evidence is clear about the standards being covered
- check that the signatory can be contacted for authentication of the validation letter, if necessary.

An example of a letter of validation is provided in Figure 3.4.

### Use of simulations

Any source of performance evidence other than the learner's normal, naturally-occurring work activity can be thought of as a simulation. However, before the learner decides to use simulation, all other sources of evidence should be examined to ensure that simulation is the most cost-effective and appropriate method.

Care must be taken to ensure that any simulated assessment meets the full requirements of the outcomes or competencies being assessed. The adviser must be confident that any competence demonstrated during the simulation can be

Your name: _____    Your identification no: _____

Organization: _____    Your adviser is: _____

### 1. What is my strategy for learning?

*After examining the criteria to be achieved, you could seek relevant information at the library or have a discussion with a colleague at work or with a mentor. Keep a record of what you do as this could count as part of the evidence you present in your portfolio.*

### 2. What have I learned?

*Based on the information you gained from the above activities, you will need to identify the knowledge you have gained, and indicate how it relates to the criteria to be assessed.*

### 3. How will I apply this knowledge?

*State how the knowledge gained will be applied to your field of study or occupation. For example, you may use it to solve an existing problem or you could describe how it might be used to solve a potential problem.*

### 4. What evidence can I demonstrate?

*List the possible sources of evidence which demonstrate you have the appropriate knowledge for each of the criteria against which you are being assessed. For example; a record of the reading you have undertaken, a copy of any notes you have made, any certificates of attendance you have obtained at training sessions. Don't forget to place a copy of any learning diaries you have completed in your portfolio!*

### 5. APL adviser comments

*The APL adviser will need to record whether he/she agrees that you have the necessary supporting knowledge, and understanding and confirm the outcomes or competencies to which this relates. The APL adviser will do this by countersigning this form and making any appropriate comments. These records should be placed in your portfolio.*

Your signature: _____    Date: _____

Signature of adviser: _____    Date: _____

**Figure 3.3** A sample learning diary (adapted from Day, 1996, and Day and Zakos, 1999)

---

**Learner's name:** *Fred Smith*          **Learner's identification no:** *00001*

**1. Declaration:**
*I have read and understood the outcomes/competencies required and I am able to state that the above individual can meet the following requirements:*

Competence/Outcomes: *Health and Safety Unit One*
Competencies/Criteria: *1a, 1b and 1c*

**2. Evidence to support the above statement, i.e. *I am able to state this because...***
*Fred looked after me when I cut my hand at work. He laid me flat, raised my hand in the air and applied a firm bandage to control the bleeding. He covered me with a blanket and told me not to eat or drink anything and then arranged an ambulance to get me to hospital. When I returned to work the next day, Fred helped me fill out the accident report book. Fred was calm throughout the incident and I really felt safe and reassured by him.*

**3. Details of person signing the letter of validation.**

Name: *Joan Smith*                    Designation: *Shop floor worker*

Qualifications: *Body Shop Operative*          Telephone: *Extension 242*

Relationship of witness to learner: *Client:*    E-mail:

Address: *The Body Shop, Peabody International*      Telephone no: *Ext. 242*

**Your signature:** _____

Date: _____

**Signature of verifier:** _____

Date: _____

NB You may be contacted by an APL assessor to confirm your observations/ comments.

---

**Figure 3.4** A sample validation letter (adapted from Day, 1996, and Day and Zakos, 1999)

transferred to the work environment and is therefore a realistic representation of the knowledge and performance/competence required.

Simulation could be used when there are issues relating to confidentiality and safety or to increase access to assessment. Some examples are:

- future requirements such as new technologies and work practices at the individual's workplace that do not offer opportunities to provide appropriate evidence
- infrequent events such as an annual inventory or the outcome of a five-year business plan, if waiting for the event to occur could delay assessment
- avoiding risks to the individual or others in the work environment, e.g. cleaning procedures in cases of chemical contamination
- procedures which may have complicated or dangerous consequences, e.g. testing for and repairing a gas leak
- life-threatening conditions, such as resuscitation of a person who has stopped breathing
- situations in which collecting evidence would intrude on personal privacy or confidentiality.

Simulations allow the learner to develop and practise skills in a safe environment and can provide useful opportunities for developmental assessment and feedback. However, when simulations are used for assessing competence against a standard, they must be set up to reflect real activities and conditions. All simulations must provide for valid and reliable assessment of the required outcomes and criteria. When planning to use a simulation, the adviser and the learner should consider the following questions:

- What arrangements have been made for identifying sources of evidence, e.g. workplace, work placement simulation at the evidence planning stage?
- When workplace evidence is not available, have opportunities to use work placements and job rotation been fully explored?
- Do other faculty/staff or assessors share a common understanding of simulation?
- What systems, processes and design criteria are in place to support the development and design of simulations?
- Are the simulations cost-effective when compared to other methods of generating and gathering evidence?
- What arrangements have been made for briefing those who are to be assessed through simulation?

### Agreeing to and reviewing an action plan for demonstration of prior learning

Learners might think that they already have the necessary knowledge and experience required to demonstrate that they can meet some of the outcomes or competencies of a programme. Much of the evidence that can be used for this has already been discussed and includes certificates and transcripts, from previous courses, work records and products, and letters of validation.

Some organizations keep a comprehensive account of staff training activities and they regularly carry out staff performance reviews. Other organizations issue workers with a personal handbook which records comments from supervisors on their performance at work. The outcomes of these staff development activities may be used as evidence, provided they relate to the criteria being assessed and they can be substantiated.

Learners may find that they can organize evidence to demonstrate several outcomes or competencies at the same time. If the assessment process is to be meaningful, it is important to consider the possibility of using this whole or 'holistic' approach to APL, rather than reducing the process to a series of unconnected observations and tasks. In doing this advisers will find that:

- the process will become more interesting
- evidence will become more meaningful and efficient
- it will avoid unnecessary repetition
- use of learners' achievements will be maximized
- it will save valuable time and energy which can be applied elsewhere.

Learners will need to take into account the way in which they organize their work and/or learning in order to make best use of the evidence they are generating. One way of doing this is to build up a portfolio of learning and experience. This process can be initiated by undertaking a self-assessment of one's current skills, abilities and competencies. The results of this activity and any supporting evidence can be included in a portfolio.

### Help the individual to prepare and present evidence for assessment

Evidence of prior learning can be collected in a portfolio. A portfolio is a record, kept in a binder, a file or a folder, of an individual's prior learning achievements – what she or he knows and can do. Some portfolios are extremely comprehensive and wide-ranging, some are more narrowly and specifically focused, depending on the purposes, objectives and goals of the learner.

### SUMMARY

This chapter has examined in detail the role of the APL practitioner, drawing upon newly emerging benchmarks for practice in order to clarify the role of the APL adviser and assessor. The key purpose, functions and activities of the APL practitioner have been outlined, and the factors which might influence the APL practitioner role have been discussed. Finally, the use of direct versus indirect evidence of prior learning has been discussed, using a portfolio approach.

While portfolios often contain many of the elements and components outlined within this chapter, there is no single 'right' way to organize and present a portfolio. In fact, people exercise a great deal of creativity in this regard. Chapter 4 examines the process of portfolio development in more detail and includes an example of an integrated approach towards portfolio development within the field of health care. In particular, it demonstrates, through case study, how the practice of APL is being implemented within colleges, universities, and the professions. Examples are drawn from the USA, UK and Canada.

 **Key learning activity 9**

Consider the sample documentation presented in this chapter.

Discuss with your co-ordinator, or a respected colleague, how relevant these are to your own organization?

How might they be improved or adapted for your own use?

Don't forget to record your discussions in your learning diary (Appendix 2).

# 4 THE PRACTICE OF APL IN COLLEGES, UNIVERSITIES AND THE PROFESSIONS

The previous chapter examined in detail the role of the APL practitioner. In particular it drew upon newly emerging benchmarks for APL practice (Appendix 1) to clarify the role of the APL adviser and assessor. This chapter identifies, through case study, how the practice of APL is being implemented within colleges, universities and the professions. Examples are drawn from the USA, UK and Canada.

- The first case study, from the USA, describes a *developmental* approach towards APL. It draws upon the principles and procedures first identified by CAEL in the 1970s and 1980s. Students are encouraged to write personal competency statements based on their prior learning. They match these personal competency statements against course outcomes in order to gain access, advanced standing or college credit.
- In the second case study, from the UK, a *credit exchange* approach towards APL is described, where students work towards the accumulation of academic credits or 'points', within a nationally-agreed credit-based system. Depending on the number of points or units accumulated, the student may gain access to, or advanced standing within, a degree programme. Students also develop a portfolio of evidence against nationally-agreed standards for practice, which are determined by professional and statutory bodies. Thus, evidence within the portfolio is used in a *complementary* way to gain both academic credit *and* professional licensure.
- In the third case study, from Canada, candidates are required to generate evidence from the workplace against nationally-agreed standards for practice, which are determined by the professional body. Evidence is collected within a portfolio and used to demonstrate continuing competence to practise. The portfolio *may* or *may not* be submitted for college credit. Thus evidence of prior learning is used in a *complementary* way to demonstrate evidence of life-long learning, as well as academic ability.

At the end of this chapter, you will have gained a greater appreciation of the diversity and context for practice, as well as external factors which might influence and shape APL policy and procedure. In particular, you will be able to:

- identify the essential features of *developmental* and *credit-based* approaches to APL
- compare and contrast these two approaches in order to identify the relative benefits of either

- indicate how best principles from either approach might be utilized in order to accommodate the needs of learners, academic institutions and the professions.

---

## USA: A DEVELOPMENTAL APPROACH

### North East State Community College

This college is located within an urban inner-city area in a north eastern state in the USA. It is a comprehensive two-year community college offering higher education in a diverse range of over 2,000 university parallel, technical and career courses to nearly 20,000 students in 101 academic disciplines. The college is the largest single-campus community college within the state, and one of the twenty largest in the USA. It has six degree granting academic divisions: Allied Health, Business Technologies, Engineering and Industrial Technologies, Extended Learning and Human Services, Fine Performing Arts and Liberal Arts and Science.

Students at the college benefit from a property tax levy agreed by the voters of the county in which it is located, which was renewed in 1998. Because of this levy, the college is able to offer high quality education at low tuition rates to the maximum amount of people in the community. The average age of a student at the college is 35 years old. Fifty-three per cent of the student population is 25 years or older. The average class size is twenty.

Part of the college's stated mission is to:

'provide quality instruction, educational activities, counselling, support services, and assessment tools to facilitate the growth and development of life-long learning and to assist individuals to achieve personal and professional goals.'

and to:

'prepare today's workforce to meet the needs of a rapidly changing technologically advanced, global economy through traditional and non-traditional alternatives.'

The college has been offering college credit for prior learning for over 24 years. It does this via an integrated programme, which serves as a model of excellence for institutions within the USA and Canada. The strengths of the programme have been recognized by the North Central Accrediting Agency. In 1991 the college received an Institutional Award from CAEL.

The Experienced Based Education Department (EBE) has responsibility for co-ordinating assessment across all academic divisions within the college. It does this through the Academic Credit Assessment Information Centre (ACAIC) and the Credit for Lifelong Learning Program (CLLP). The ACAIC was established in

1983 to co-ordinate other activities at the college, e.g. articulation agreements[1]. This case study will centre upon the work of the CLLP.

The CLLP has been in existence since 1976. It was developed as a result of increased faculty interest in serving the needs of adult learners, and an increased growth in non-traditional learning activities. For example, in a recent CAEL study, *Best Practices in Adult Learning* (1999), it is reported that curriculum strategy at the college includes engaging learners as full partners in the education process, offering as many options for learning as possible, assisting learners in forming and participating in collaborative learning activities and defining roles of learning facilitators by the needs of the learners.

Within the CLLP, students prepare portfolios which describe and document their prior learning against specific courses at the college. Students are guided by EBE staff through the process of identifying college level learning, matching their learning to specific courses and documenting that learning. The portfolios are evaluated by faculty members from academic departments, who have been specifically prepared to undertake a role. The quality assurance of portfolios is undertaken by the EBE department, a cross-faculty service.

The college identifies the strengths of the CLLP: involvement of academic faculty in the award of academic credit and choice of assessment method; the diverse number of assessment options available; integration of APL into the institution; and the college's commitment to expanding access to all learners. Policy and practice within the CLLP draws heavily on literature from the field of humanistic adult learning (see Chapter 1) as well as CAEL's early work on assessment of work-based and experiential learning (Chapter 1).

CLLP uses a portfolio approach towards assessment. The college defines the portfolio, both in terms of a product and a process:

> 'A portfolio is a written document or record used as a vehicle for organizing and distilling raw prior learning experiences and accomplishments into a manageable form for assessment of college-level learning. Portfolio is also a term that has come to represent the entire process by which learning from prior experiences can be translated into educational outcomes or competencies, documented and assessed for academic credit. It is not unusual to hear a faculty tell a student: You should portfolio that course.'

Access to CLLP is via the EBE 100 course. This is an eleven-week programme delivered via the classroom, television, video cassette or the Internet. The programme introduces the learner to the value of experiential learning, critical reflection, and the relationship of these activities to college-level learning. Students are also introduced to the policies and procedures of the college and provided with sample documentation. At the end of the EBE 100 programme,

1 Articulation agreements are formal agreements between two academic institutions detailing the recognition of credit between them, e.g. agreements with local universities which enable students to transfer from a two-year associate degree to a four-year baccalaureate programme.

the student is able to: identify his or her learning from experience; identify future academic goals that build upon his or her prior learning; match his or her learning to specific course outcomes; examine potential assessment options and possible alternatives; learn how to write a portfolio; and develop an educational plan detailing how he or she is going to complete future academic goals. On completion, students receive three credit hours for the CLLP, plus credit towards other specific courses. For example, in order to obtain an associate degree, students require 90 credit hours, depending on their field of study. Typically, on the CLLP most students achieve nine to twelve credit hours[2], some individuals have earned as much as 70 credit hours. Over 25,000 credit hours have been awarded since the programme's inception.

The EBE 100 programme utilizes an *adult-centred* approach towards learning (see Chapter 1). Through a series of carefully guided individual and group exercises, the student develops a personal portfolio which includes: a *cover letter* stating the credit requested; a *chronological record*, a year-by-year account of his or her experiences since high school; a *life history paper*, a 4–5-page paper detailing important events, turning points and insights; a *goals paper* listing personal, career and educational goals. The portfolio also contains a *competency statement* which is a concise statement of experience and how it meets course aims; plus *documentation of any learning experience* which supports the competencies identified.

CLLP accredits prior learning, not experience. To ensure this, internal policy and procedures state that prior learning outcomes should:

> 'Be measurable; Be at a level of achievement defined by the faculty; Be applicable outside the specific job or context in which it was learned; Have a knowledge base; Imply a conceptual, as well as a practical, understanding; Show some relationship to degree goals and/or lifelong learning goals.'

During the EBE 100 programme, students discuss the difference between experience and learning, comparing their personal chronological record with the course syllabus. To assist this process, students are asked to complete a *learning experience worksheet* (see Figure 4.1). This worksheet assists the student to identify, analyse and articulate prior experiential learning against specific course outcomes.

Students then draw upon this information to write one or more personal competency statements. The competency statement is: 'a narrative detailing learning from prior experience as it relates to a specific [name of college deleted] course.' (Mann 1998: 53). A competency statement is written for each course the student is hoping to gain credit for, using the matrix outlined in Table 4.1.

This approach to competency development is quite different to that used

---

2 Credit hours: the number of hours a week a student attends a given class. Three credit hours means a student attends a particular course three hours per week. If the course is passed, then three credit hours may apply towards graduation.

| Experience, e.g. | Time spent in activity | Description of duties, tasks or activities | Description of outcomes or competencies | Documentation, i.e. suggest ways in which the evaluator can judge you |
|---|---|---|---|---|
| Employment Education Volunteer Recreation Awards Publications Reading Travel | | | | |

**Figure 4.1**   A learning experience worksheet

within the credit-based model of APL, where competencies to be achieved are shaped by an external validating body, e.g. NVQs (Chapter 1).

During week 10 of the programme, EBE staff review student portfolios, prior to submission for faculty evaluation. During the review, students are prompted by EBE staff to re-evaluate the competencies they have identified, by asking the following questions:

'Have I covered the course objectives?
Have I explained my experiences clearly enough?
Have I organized my experiences and learning so that they can be easily followed?
Have I separated my learning from experience?
Am I being clear and concise?
Am I leaving too much for the evaluator to assume?
Am I repeating myself too much?'

**Table 4.1**   Identifying a competency

| Description of experience | Learning from experience | Documentation |
|---|---|---|
| Where learning took place? Length of experience ? Job title? Responsibilities of job? People supervised? Training attended? Books/articles read? Contexts and circumstances? | I learned … I acquired this knowledge through … I gained this insight … I developed the skill of … | Testimonials Certificates Commendations Job descriptions Products from work Articles published |

Assessment of portfolios is undertaken by faculty, using the marking schema outlined below.

---

### Marking schema for CLLP

**Allocation of points:**
Chronological record = 20 points
Life history = 20 points
Goals paper = 20 points
Competency = 20 points
Documentation = 10 points
EBE review of portfolio = 10 points

**Possible final grades:**
A = 90–100 points
B = 80–89 points
C = 70–79 points
D = 60–69 points
F = 59 or below

---

Close associations between the EBE department and faculty helps to prevent the phenomena of 'double counting', that is, students receiving credit for the same knowledge twice (see CAEL standards for APL, page 13). Any 'top up' learning that might be identified as a result of this assessment is achieved through an individualized learning contract between faculty and student.

The identification of a plan for continued learning is a common feature of developmental approaches towards practice. It is in sharp contrast to the credit-based approach, which confirms existing competence, or establishes an individual's position within an agreed credit framework based on their prior certificated learning.

The CLLP has been successfully running for nearly 25 years. As a consequence, policies and procedures have been fully integrated across the faculties and divisions within the college. The EBE service is, therefore, subject to the same systematic and periodic review as other disciplines within the division. This includes internal periodic review, as well as external audit by the North Central Accrediting Agency. Newly appointed faculty are invited to contact EBE staff to discuss any individual training required to support their role. Mentorship is also provided by faculty colleagues who are experienced in assessment of portfolios.

Faculty staff believe that the success of the CLLP is due to:

- a college culture which fosters and supports innovation and change
- recognition of the economic and demographic needs of the local community
- strong leadership and guidance from the Experienced Based Education service

- the seniority/credibility of faculty assessors
- mentorship and supervision at faculty level for newly appointed faculty staff
- clearly specified syllabi and curriculum outcomes
- clearly specified assessment guidelines and procedures for staff and students
- flexible methods of assessment and learning delivery.

Students report that they value the structure and the individualized support they receive on the CLLP. For example, comments regarding the programme include:

'Following the procedures taught in the portfolio development course at Sinclair, over one winter and spring I prepared portfolios for 9 courses ... and earned 27 college credits.'

'I enrolled on the EBE 100 class to determine if anything I learned on the job was equivalent to what is taught in the classroom. The EBE staff are extremely helpful, and provided a step-by-step procedure on how to document and prove what you know is worth college credit.'

An overview of the CLLP is presented in Figure 4.2.

## UK: A CREDIT-BASED APPROACH

### Northern School of Nursing and Midwifery

The school first developed APL in 1993, in response to the English National Board for Nursing, Midwifery and Health Visiting (ENB)[3] Framework for Continuing Professional Development, as the ENB required that institutions offering continuing professional development should be modularized and offer APL.

The Framework for Continuing Professional Development is incorporated within the English National Board's Higher Award. This is both a professional and academic qualification. The ENB Higher Award is based upon the following ten key characteristics:

- professional accountability and responsibility
- clinical expertise with a specific client
- use of research to plan, implement and evaluate strategies to improve care
- team working and building, and multi-disciplinary team leadership
- flexible and innovative approaches to care
- use of health promotion strategies

3 The ENB are a professional body for nurse training, responsible for conjointly approving all nurse training programmes delivered within English universities. There are also Welsh, Scottish and Northern Ireland nursing boards, which are governed by the UK statutory body for nursing, the United Kingdom Central Council for Nursing, Midwifery and Health Visiting.

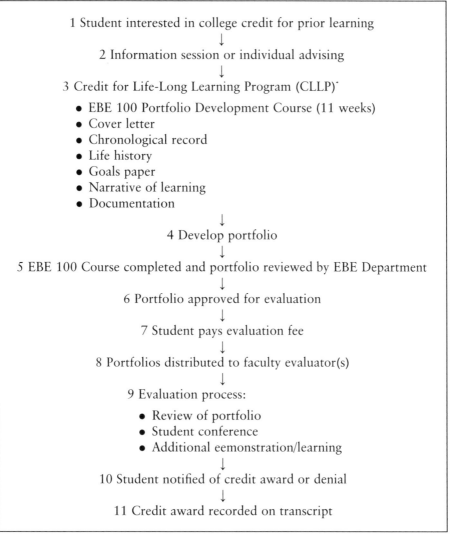

1 Student interested in college credit for prior learning
↓
2 Information session or individual advising
↓
3 Credit for Life-Long Learning Program (CLLP)˙

- EBE 100 Portfolio Development Course (11 weeks)
- Cover letter
- Chronological record
- Life history
- Goals paper
- Narrative of learning
- Documentation

↓
4 Develop portfolio
↓
5 EBE 100 Course completed and portfolio reviewed by EBE Department
↓
6 Portfolio approved for evaluation
↓
7 Student pays evaluation fee
↓
8 Portfolios distributed to faculty evaluator(s)
↓
9 Evaluation process:

- Review of portfolio
- Student conference
- Additional eemonstration/learning

↓
10 Student notified of credit award or denial
↓
11 Credit award recorded on transcript

**Figure 4.2** The Credit for Life-Long Learning Program (Mann, 1998: 9)

- facilitating and assessing development in others
- handling information and making informed clinical decisions
- setting standards and evaluating quality of care
- initiating, managing and evaluating clinical change.

These characteristics represent the areas of skill, knowledge and expertise which describe the attributes of practitioners working closely with patients and clients. They also provide a benchmark against which all practitioners can examine the range and scope of their practice. Each nurse, midwife or health visitor can reflect on the ten key characteristics and plan an individual programme of professional development related to his or her own particular area of practice.

Practitioners can also direct and integrate their continuing education activities, as each of the ten key characteristics has associated learning outcomes. They can do this in a flexible way, in partnership with educationalists and managers, to plan and negotiate learning to meet their particular needs. To do this, they are required to keep a professional portfolio which demonstrates their ability to integrate all ten key characteristics into their practice.

Practitioners who want formal recognition for their continuing education can aim for the Higher Award, and register as a student with an approved college of nursing and midwifery. The ENB Higher Award is a post-registration professional award which has been accredited at degree level. In order to achieve this award, the practitioners must demonstrate their ability to integrate all ten key characteristics into their practice. They must also achieve mastery in each of the associated learning outcomes. In achieving these learning outcomes, practitioners need to demonstrate change in their practice with a specific client group. Higher award programmes are flexible and modular. For example, they may include existing post-registration clinical courses, open learning programmes, planned work-based experience, individual work on particular topics, or courses run by a variety of organizations as long as they are relevant to the ten key characteristics.

The Higher Award incorporates a CATs scheme (Chapter 1). This means that practitioners can gain credit for learning, either from formal programmes, learning demonstrated in practice or life experiences. Because the Board's Framework and Higher Award use a modular approach to learning, practitioners can develop a highly individualized programme or can join a group.

In 1995, policies and procedures were evaluated by practitioners within the school, using a structured questionnaire. The questionnaire sought responses from candidates who were at the beginning, mid-point and end of their experience. Items for the questionnaire were based on anecdotal feedback received from previous cohorts.

As a consequence of this activity, the concerns raised by previous candidates have been addressed within newly developed guidelines. These guidelines define issues such as the validity, sufficiency, currency, relevance and authenticity of evidence and also outline local procedures and documentation (see Figure 4.3).

A glossary of assessment terms, a bibliography on APL, a taxonomy of outcomes, and how this relates to the assessment requirements of individual modules, is also given. As a result of developing these new guidelines, practitioners within the school report that less one-to-one guidance is now required, although this is still provided by telephone and personal interviews. In addition, potential students are offered guidance via 'road shows' and outreach.

Originally, the school envisaged separate schemes for accreditation of prior certificated learning and accreditation of prior experiential learning (Chapter 1). However, this proved to be unworkable since many students have both certified learning (credit exchange) and learning gained through work experience (developmental). In practice, most claims combine elements of both, and the proce-

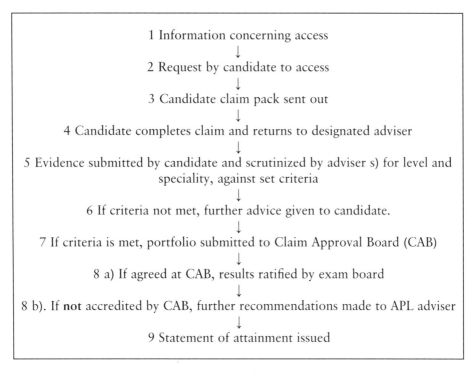

1 Information concerning access
↓
2 Request by candidate to access
↓
3 Candidate claim pack sent out
↓
4 Candidate completes claim and returns to designated adviser
↓
5 Evidence submitted by candidate and scrutinized by adviser s) for level and speciality, against set criteria
↓
6 If criteria not met, further advice given to candidate.
↓
7 If criteria is met, portfolio submitted to Claim Approval Board (CAB)
↓
8 a) If agreed at CAB, results ratified by exam board
↓
8 b). If **not** accredited by CAB, further recommendations made to APL adviser
↓
9 Statement of attainment issued

**Figure 4.3** The APL process at the Northern School of Nursing and Midwifery

dures are the same for both certificated and experiential learning. However, university regulations make a distinction between prior certificated learning and prior experiential learning, particularly when considering currency of evidence. Therefore claims for prior certificated learning in excess of five years old are required to be supported by recent experiential learning which demonstrates that this prior knowledge has been recently applied to practice.

Clearly, within this organization the distinction between credit exchange and developmental approaches towards APL is no longer applicable, rather best principles from both are being applied in a complementary way to meet the needs of the learner, as well as the university's demands for accreditation.

APL within the school is used for access, advanced standing and credit. It is targeted towards the continuing professional development of practising nurses, particularly the Diploma in Professional Nursing Practice (Level 2 credits) and the B.Sc. in Professional Nursing Practice (Level 3 credits)[4].

4 Within the UK, a national credit and accumulation transfer system (CATs) is in place for academic qualifications, as well as NVQs. In order to obtain a degree, the student must achieve 120 credits at level 1 (certificate), plus 120 credits at level 2 (diploma), plus 120 credits at level 3 (degree). A degree is awarded if 360 credits are achieved by the student.

The roles of adviser and assessor are separated within the school. Students submit their claim via a portfolio. Evidence contained within the portfolio must be verified by a professional colleague. The portfolio is initially scrutinized by an adviser for currency, sufficiency, etc. The portfolio is then passed to a specialist nurse teacher, who makes an assessment of specialist clinical evidence, using assessment guidelines agreed within the school.

The specialist assessors make a written report and the claim, together with the evidence and assessors' reports, are sent to the Claims Approval Board (CAB). The CAB consists of all advisers within the school, as well as the co-ordinator. The CAB reviews all claims in detail and discusses any questions or differences of opinion. Claims are either accepted or referred back to the student, for example, in one CAB meeting at which 33 B.Sc. candidates submitted claims, three were referred back.

If there is an element of doubt about the nature of the evidence presented, the CAB may recommend that the student do further work or undertake a *viva voice*. If the student has not undertaken academic work for some time, then at least one written piece of evidence is required. More experienced students are often examined through *viva voice*. The university, not the school, limits credits to two-thirds of an academic award.

All claims are sampled annually by external examiners who are jointly appointed by the university and the ENB, as well as the Faculty Chair of the Undergraduate Studies Committee. The work of the CAB is seen as an important process for maintaining the quality of assessment, and the continuing development of practitioners, who are continuously asked to reflect upon, and justify, their assessment decisions. In this way consistency of assessment can be maintained across the school and its outreach centres.

## CANADA: A COMPLEMENTARY APPROACH

### The Canadian Technology Human Resources Board (CTHRB)

The CTHRB, through the 'Technofile' project have established on-line Canadian Technology Standards (CTS) which are based on standards required for competent performance in the workplace. These can be assessed and validated by the CTHRB to ensure that individuals perform at work to nationally-agreed standards. Assessment for validation is free from any unnecessary barriers which might restrict access, and available to all those who are able to reach the required standard, by whatever means. The assessment system developed for the CTHRB framework is designed to meet the technology industry's needs for reliability and consistency in assessing the competence of technicians and technologists. It is underpinned by the following principles (Day and Zakos, 1999):

- *Relevance*: assessment of individual competence is against the standards laid down by the CTHRB, and is based upon individual career development needs. Individuals who are assessed as being competent are therefore considered to be employable in their chosen field of technology

- *Flexibility*: it is acknowledged that the unique way in which an individual responds and adapts to their learning environment is an essential part of the assessment process. The growing number of people with specific needs who will be accessing the CTHRB framework will mean that a diverse and individualized approach towards assessment needs to be undertaken
- *Integrity*: in order to maintain the unique status of the technology professions in Canada, all stakeholders must be convinced that the assessment process is accessible, transparent, rigorous and credible. To this end a systematic approach to ensure the quality of the assessment process has been developed
- *Utility*: the assessment process should be efficient, straightforward, free from any unnecessary jargon and user-friendly. It should meet the needs of the learner and the requirements of the CTHRB, without overburdening the resources of the approved CTS validating agent.

Within the CTHRB framework, emphasis is placed upon the achievement of recognized learning outcomes. The way in which these outcomes are achieved is not specified because it is acknowledged that individuals will learn at different speeds or develop skills and knowledge at different times. Experienced people are given credit for their prior learning, including credit for previous learning obtained in education and employment, as well as competence gained in unpaid work.

Within the CTHRB framework, assessment is available to all individuals who have the potential to achieve the required standard. Therefore assessment is not dependent upon a particular mode of learning, location of learning, upper or lower age limits or on any actions which require candidates to spend a specified period of time in education, training or work.

Validation of competence by the CTHRB is achieved by assessing the candidate against nationally-agreed Canadian Technology Standards. These include technical skills, planning and problem-solving skills, the ability to deal with unexpected events, i.e. contingencies, the ability to work with other people, and the ability to apply relevant knowledge to competent performance

Evidence to indicate that these standards can be achieved is divided into: *performance evidence* and *knowledge evidence*. There are two types of performance evidence:

- *products of the candidate's work* – items which the candidate has produced or worked on, documents produced as part of a work activity, and so on. The evidence may be in the form of the product itself, or may be a record or photograph of the product
- *evidence of the way the candidate carried out activities* – evidence of the processes involved in demonstrating competence. This often takes the form of letters of validation, assessor observation, authenticated reports of the candidate undertaking the activity, or audio or video recordings of the candidate's work.

Within the CTHRB framework, *knowledge* and *understanding* are integral to competent performance; they are not something separate from it. Evidence of an individual's knowledge can be drawn from formal written and oral tests, or from informal questioning, and can be inferred directly from performance. Knowledge is about knowing what should be done, how it should be done, why it should be done and what should be done if circumstances change. It includes knowledge of facts and procedures, understanding of theories and principles, and ways of using and applying knowledge. Knowledge evidence also helps to predict whether a candidate will be able to perform competently in new settings and cope with new problems. Although knowledge can be inferred through competent performance, the CTHRB recognize it is unlikely that this will satisfy all the requirements of the standard being assessed. In which case, questioning in the workplace or written tests are used as a more suitable means of checking the breadth and depth of an individual's knowledge. Assessors judge the best mix of knowledge evidence according to individual circumstances and the standard being assessed.

In undertaking assessment, candidates and assessors collaborate in order to minimize the volume of evidence required. Candidates familiarize themselves with the requirements of the CTHRB framework and the Canadian Technology Standards. Copies of the relevant technology standards are available to candidates 'on line'. Candidates are encouraged to:

- make a self-assessment of their own competence
- request formal assessment
- identify opportunities for evidence collection
- decide how to present evidence
- arrange observation by supervisors
- collect witness testimony from colleagues
- identify suitable ways of meeting their own continuing development needs.

Responsibility for managing assessment planning rests with the assessor, supported and advised by the centre co-ordinator. The assessor's role in assessment planning includes:

- one-to-one discussions with the candidate
- discussions with the centre co-ordinator
- making decisions on the type of evidence needed
- identifying opportunities for evidence collection
- making arrangements for judging evidence
- making arrangements for reviewing the candidate's progress and their assessment plan.

Many candidates already have some evidence of their competence to practise. In which case the candidate's assessor helps the candidate to:

- identify relevant achievements, including those from work and unpaid work
- agree and review an action plan for assessment
- help prepare and present evidence for assessment.

The CTHRB use a systematic approach towards assessment planning. This includes the following steps:

1 Identify evidence which might exist from other credentials, products or records which have already been produced by the candidate.
2 Compare this evidence against each of the competence statements outlined in the Canadian Technology Standards to determine a possible fit. Identify any gaps or mismatches.
3 From the gaps identified, find any competencies which might occur naturally, and plan appropriate opportunities to demonstrate the candidate's ability to perform these, e.g. from the candidate's everyday work or from a temporary placement in a different job role.
4 Identify any competencies which might not occur naturally. Plan alternative ways to collect evidence relating to these, e.g. simulations or case studies, projects, etc.
5 Identify other forms of assessment to fully cover knowledge and under-standing not demonstrated through performance, e.g. discussion, questioning, reflective accounts, written tests, etc.

The CTHRB framework gives individuals an opportunity to gain validation for the experience and skills developed through activities outside the workplace. In doing this, the CTHRB utilize a candidate-led approach, which can be particu-larly appropriate if it is difficult for the assessor to carry out direct observation of the candidate's performance. In particular, this approach:

• helps to reduce an assessor's workload
• helps to promote a candidate's involvement in their own assessment
• helps to enhance self-assessment skills
• helps candidates to identify their own specific learning needs
• makes it easier for candidates to identify opportunities which the assessor may miss.

In using this approach, the assessor establishes whether items of evidence are good enough to be taken into account when making an assessment decision. In particular the assessor checks that the evidence is valid and directly relates to the competencies outlined in the national technology standards. The assessor also checks to see if the evidence meets each of the specifications outlined within the standards, for example, contingencies and knowledge component.

Finally, the assessor checks that the evidence is authentic and is the candi-date's own work. Often it is necessary for the assessor to carry out questioning, or for the candidate to collect further performance evidence in order to confirm that evidence is authentic. For example, when looking at a computer printout, it can be difficult to tell if an item of evidence is entirely the candidate's own work, or it may be difficult to differentiate the candidate's own work from that produced by others in his or her work team.

Once each item of evidence has been collected, the assessor judges whether or not the candidate is competent. Sufficiency becomes a key issue at this stage – the assessor has to decide whether there is sufficient evidence to demonstrate that a candidate is competent. Within the CTHRB framework, sufficiency is achieved if the candidate's evidence is considered to be current and up-to-date, if the candidate's performance is consistent and can be demonstrated over a period of time, and also, if the candidate can demonstrate that he or she has the relevant knowledge and understanding, and can apply it to their occupation. From the CTHRB's point of view, competence is about being able to perform to the standard required in employment. It would be unsafe to infer that a candidate can perform to the national standard solely on the basis of their knowledge and understanding. Therefore evidence must demonstrate that the candidate can actually use this knowledge and understanding under workplace conditions to meet the performance outlined within the technology standards.

Within the CTHRB framework, the amount of evidence required to confirm competence depends on a number of factors, including the specific requirements of the competence being assessed and the opportunities open to the candidate to collect evidence. An absolute minimum would be to have one item of evidence, provided this met each of the criteria outlined within the competence statement. However, in practice a single item of evidence is unlikely to demonstrate a candidate's ability to perform consistently. A number of items collected over a period of time would be needed to demonstrate this. An evidence log is used for this purpose, so that candidates can keep a daily record of products and processes relating to the national standards.

Within the CTHRB framework, if assessors are unsure about the depth of knowledge required, they clarify this with their centre co-ordinator. Centre co-ordinators hold standardization meetings for this purpose. At these meetings, the assessment team reach a common agreement and understanding about the nature of knowledge and performance evidence. In this way, consistency of assessment is achieved across the centre.

Candidates may include evidence from prior learning in their overall package of evidence. This will have been checked at the judging stage for validity and authenticity. However, it is important to recognize that even if evidence meets the standard, the candidate may not be currently competent if it was produced some years ago. It is essential that a candidate's evidence shows current competence. If the assessor is not a 100 per cent sure of this, it may be necessary to include a more recent piece of performance evidence in the overall package. The centre co-ordinator advises on this issue.

The CTHRB estimates that around 100,000 technicians and technologists across Canada are eligible for assessment against the Canadian Technology Standards. Quality is the key to the success of the CTHRB framework. It is the responsibility of all those who are involved in the CTS assessment process, i.e. candidates, assessor, centre co-ordinators and the CTHRB. Only those organizations who meet the CTHRB quality seal of approval are allowed to validate the outcomes of assessment. Those involved in assessment include:

- *Candidates*: individuals seeking credit for their competence by showing that they can perform to Canadian Technology Standards by demonstrating the specified knowledge, understanding and skills required. Candidates are responsible for the quality of evidence they provide to assessors.
- *Assessors*: individuals who have sufficient occupational expertise to be able to make accurate assessment decisions in the areas for which they are responsible. They are appointed by an approved validating agent to assess candidate evidence. Assessors are in direct contact with candidates. They judge candidate evidence against CTHRB Canadian Technology Standards. They decide whether the candidate has demonstrated competence. They ensure that their own assessment practice meets CTHRB requirements.
- *Centre co-ordinators*: individuals who can demonstrate specific competence in assessment. They understand the structure of the standards relating to each assessment and are able to draw upon sufficient occupational expertise, to be able to authenticate assessment decisions made by assessors. Centre co-ordinators are appointed by an approved validating agent to ensure the consistency and quality of assessment within the agency. They work with assessors to assure the quality and consistency of assessment. They sample candidate assessments to ensure consistency and make sure that assessment records and documents meet the aims of the agency and the requirements of the CTHRB. They also ensure that requests for validation are based on assessments which are of consistent quality. Centre co-ordinators provide support and guidance for assessors and act as a contact for the CTHRB and the external adviser. They request candidate validation from the CTHRB.
- *Approved validating agents*: organizations approved by the CTHRB to assess individual competence against Canadian Technology Standards. These organizations manage assessment on a day-to-day basis. They have effective assessment practices and quality assurance procedures and meet CTHRB requirements for validation of competence, against Canadian Technology Standards. Validating agents have sufficient competent centre co-ordinators and assessors with enough time and authority to carry out their roles effectively.
- *External advisers*: individuals who have competencies which qualify them to perform the duties of an external adviser. They understand the structure of the standards relating to each assessment and are able to draw upon sufficient occupational expertise, to be able to authenticate assessment decisions made by assessors. They are appointed by the CTHRB to monitor the work of approved validating agents. They are the key link between the CTHRB and the approved agency and ensures that assessment decisions are consistent across agencies. External advisers ensure that the quality of assessment meets CTHRB requirements. They sample candidate assessments and monitor assessment practice in approved agencies. They make regular visits to agencies and assessment locations in order to provide feedback on assessment practice.
- *CTHRB*: the Canadian Technology Human Resources Board develops and validates Canadian Technology Standards on behalf of the technology

professions in Canada. It ensures quality and consistency of assessment for validation. It produces guidance for approved validating agents. The CTHRB appoints, supports and develops external advisers, allocates them to validating agents and monitors their work. The CTHRB approves and monitors validating agents against validating agent approval criteria. It collects information from agencies to make informed decisions about the delivery of Canadian Technology Standards.

 **Key learning activity 10**

Select one of the case studies presented in this chapter, and answer the following questions.

1   How have the fundamentals of a credit-based system been met?
2   How has rigorous assessment been maintained ?
3   What is the role of the APL adviser?
4   How does this role differ from the APL assessor?
5   How is any potential conflict of interest avoided during the assessment process?
6   What improvements (if any) could be made to both policy and procedure?

Now consider each of the case studies and answer the following questions.

7   What is the difference between the way in which competencies or learning outcomes are derived within the US, Canadian and UK case studies?
8   How might this difference influence the practice of APL?

Don't forget to record your answers in your learning diary.

 **Key learning activity 11**

Using the guidelines outlined in Chapter 5, obtain and critically read:

Butterworth, C. (1992) More than one bite at the APEL: contrasting models of accrediting prior learning. *Journal of Further and Higher Education*. Vol. 16, No. 3, pp 39–51.

Discuss the article with your co-ordinator, or a respected colleague. Don't forget to use your learning diary to record your ideas and reactions.

SUMMARY

This chapter has examined policy and practice within colleges, universities and the professions. Examples from Canada, the UK and the US have been presented. Although policy and practice can appear to be diverse, and may be often be context-specific, it is more often than not underpinned by the following principles.

---

### Principles underpinning an APL strategy

- The use of an eclectic model for assessment in order to accommodate both institutional and professional body requirements for academic credit and licensure
- Diverse and learner-centred assessment methods, using a portfolio approach
- Flexible curriculum, i.e. modularized, with possibilities for individual specialization, as well as continued life-long learning
- Clear and explicit curriculum levels and outcomes
- Assessment of learning and not experience
- Clear and explicit assessment processes, e.g. guidelines for both candidates and practitioners
- Clear and explicit roles and procedures, e.g. for the adviser and assessor
- Separation of adviser and assessor function to minimize assessment bias
- Continuous quality control, e.g. verification by faculty committee, or the provision of a cross-faculty service
- Continuing development of learners, advisers and assessors

---

The next chapter is designed to assist you in the development of your own portfolio, so that your continuing competence to practise can be affirmed and your personal development needs can be addressed.

# 5 A COMPLEMENTARY APPROACH

The previous chapter examined the practice of APL in diverse situations, and within different cultures, and identified common principles which underpin an APL strategy (page 71). A significant finding has emerged from this overview, namely, a move away from credit-based and developmental models of practice, towards a more *complementary* approach. This chapter examines in more detail the complementary approach towards APL.

The complementary approach towards assessment of prior learning attempts to combine best practice from credit-based and developmental models by ensuring that evidence of prior learning is not only relevant to an individual's ongoing life experience, but also meets the demands of rigorous assessment (page 6). Key to this process is the development of a portfolio – in this chapter, two examples from the field of health care are presented.

At the end of this chapter, you will be able to:

- organize and develop a portfolio; either for professional recognition, and/or academic credit
- discuss how portfolio evidence might meet the demands of *validity, reliability, sufficiency, currency* and *authenticity*.

## THE COMPLEMENTARY APPROACH TOWARDS APL PRACTICE

Within the complementary approach evidence of prior learning, often contained within a portfolio, is not only used for the purpose of access, advanced standing or academic credit, but is also used for the purpose of continuing personal or professional development. This is entirely consistent with CAPLA's view of the practitioner's role, which is to:

> *review progress and/or assess achievements, so that individuals and organizations can achieve their personal development and/or education and training objectives.*

Day (2000)

## THE PORTFOLIO PROCESS

The portfolio process draws upon the strengths of peer learning as well as individual analysis. It often involves a series of activities and exercises designed to help learners identify, describe and provide evidence of what they know and can do. Some of these exercises focus upon enabling the learner to become more conscious and specific about the breadth, depth and nature of their own learning. Others prompt the learner to think critically and creatively about their goals and objectives. Still others emphasize the process of gathering and presenting credible and sufficient evidence to substantiate the learning claims the individual is presenting. Whether working with an individual or group, the tasks of an adviser are basically threefold, to enable individuals to:

- identify and describe relevant learning
- develop and present examples of prior learning achievements
- document, organize and present a comprehensive, coherent and credible account of their prior learning.

Some of the exercises and activities used by the adviser may include the systematic development of a life chronology. This helps trigger memories of the many events and settings an individual has experienced and often leads to an in-depth analysis and identification of the learning that took place in those settings. A summary life history paper helps individuals capture those aspects of their life and learning that are most significant to them.

A learning narrative may also be used. This is a detailed examination of a particular event or experience in which the crucial distinction between the *experience* and the *learning* that occurred is emphasized. Initially many people find this a difficult distinction to make: learning always takes place in a experiential setting but the learning is not the same as the experience. For prior learning to be recognized, it must be measurable, at a level of achievement defined by the faculty, and applicable outside the specific job or context in which it was learned. It must also have a knowledge base, imply a conceptual, as well as a practical, understanding and show some relationship to degree goals and/or life-long learning goals.

## The contents of a portfolio

Individuals may develop a portfolio for a variety of reasons. For example, it may be for a specific purpose such as gaining admission or advanced standing to a programme of further education and training or continuing employment or re-licensure in a particular field or profession. In these instances, the portfolio will contain a record of the learner's personal development which has been built up over a period of time. This will often include:

- any plans the learner has made for his or her ongoing learning
- a review of the learner's actions since commencing activities
- descriptions of any learning activities undertaken at work or place of study
- evidence from others about the learner's skills and abilities.

The way in which a learner presents his or her portfolio is crucial. It should be easy to follow. The adviser should also be able to readily identify any learning that has taken place and any evidence of the learner's claim of competence. There should be a contents page which outlines each section of the portfolio.

Each section of the portfolio should represent a competency or outcome and its associated criteria.

Within each section, the learner should place the evidence he or she has collected – this should be complete, signed, dated and appropriately cross-referenced to the contents page (this could be done numerically or with colour codes). Each section should then be prefaced by a brief summary of its content. A portfolio submitted for academic credit may be rejected if it is poorly presented, so it is important to make sure that the learner's name is clearly written on it, that documents and records are legible and signed and the portfolio is neatly packaged and organized.

## Developing a portfolio

Probably one of the most difficult tasks for the learner is deciding what to include in a portfolio. The possible sources of evidence that might be used have already been discussed. However, the art of building a portfolio is a learning process in itself, which develops self-reflection and critical thinking skills. Although highly individualized, portfolio development is often successfully accomplished in small groups. Adult learners work closely with each other to identify and document significant learning events in their lives assisted by a facilitator skilled in interpersonal communication, group dynamics and adult learning principles. The development of a portfolio is a continuous and reflective process. It includes the following stages:

1  Familiarization with any outcomes or competencies required
2  Review of existing abilities and prior achievements
3  Self-assessment and production of a personal profile
4  Identification of any personal development needs, e.g. any 'top-up' learning that is needed
5  Identification of other sources of help and guidance
6  Identification of other appropriate sources of evidence
7  Identification of opportunities to maximize evidence generation
8  Planning and organizing assessments
9  Compiling the evidence.

## Appraising the portfolio

Evidence in the portfolio should be: *valid* and *relevant* to any personal, professional or academic outcomes or competencies for which the learner is seeking recognition or credit; *sufficient* to meet all of the criteria required; *authentic* and be the learner's own work; *current* or up-to-date; and able to demonstrate that the learner has developed appropriate knowledge and understanding.

### Validity

It would be inaccurate to infer that the learner was competent on the basis of his or her knowledge alone. Any evidence must also demonstrate that the learner can actually use and apply his or her skills and knowledge to meet the required criteria. The amount of evidence required will depend on a number of factors, including the specific requirements of the outcome or competence being appraised, as well as the opportunities open to the learner to collect evidence. Collecting several diverse pieces of evidence relating to the knowledge and skills required of a competency or an outcome can strengthen the validity of the evidence the learner presents. Similarly, several letters of validation gathered from colleagues, clients and supervisors about the learner's skills and abilities will provide evidence of different dimensions of the learner's work. This is called *triangulation* – using a variety of diverse sources of evidence to demonstrate competence.

## Sufficiency

Sufficiency as been achieved if the learner meets all of the criteria within each outcome or competence that is required; can demonstrate that the evidence is current and up-to-date; is consistent with his or her performance and can be demonstrated over a period of time; and can demonstrate that he or she has relevant knowledge and understanding and can apply this. An absolute minimum would be to have one item of evidence, provided it met each of the criteria outlined within the outcome or competency required. However, in practice, a single item of evidence is unlikely to demonstrate the learner's ability to perform consistently. A number of items collected over a period of time would be needed to demonstrate this. An evidence log can be useful for this purpose.

## Authenticity

It is important to be certain that all of the evidence is the learner's own work. For example, when looking at a computer printout, it can be difficult to tell if an item of evidence is entirely the individual's own work or whether it was produced by the learner as a member of a work team. In these cases, a letter of validation could confirm the authenticity of evidence which is being put forward by the learner.

## Currency

The learner will include evidence from prior learning related to specific competences in his or her portfolio. This should be checked by the adviser for validity and authenticity. It is important to recognize that even if the evidence meets the required criteria, it may not demonstrate that the learner is currently competent if it was produced some years ago. It is essential that the learner's evidence shows current competence. If the adviser is not 100 per cent sure of this, it may be necessary to seek further advice from faculty or for the learner to include a more recent piece of evidence in his or her portfolio.

## Underpinning knowledge and understanding

Knowledge and understanding are critical to competent performance. The learner must be able to demonstrate that he or she has any appropriate supporting knowledge and understanding listed in each outcome or competence statement. The learner can do this through written and oral questioning or demonstrate this through his/her performance. However, it is unlikely that performance evidence alone will be sufficient. Therefore, a combination of evidence might be used, e.g. written and oral questioning, plus direct observation of performance. If the adviser is unsure about the depth of knowledge required, he or she can check this with a respected colleague or with a faculty member. Standardization meetings are useful for this purpose. At these meetings, the assessment team can reach a common agreement and understanding about the nature of knowledge and performance evidence. In this way consistency can be achieved.

## USE OF PORTFOLIOS IN CONTINUING PROFESSIONAL DEVELOPMENT PROGRAMMES

### Canada: British Columbia College of Pharmacy CARE Programme

The College of Pharmacists in British Columbia recognizes the national and worldwide movement towards self-directed learning, public demand for high standards of health care and the governmental mandate for ongoing quality assurance. To support this, the College of Pharmacists has implemented a professional development programme which is based upon:

- *a practice review and audit*: Practitioners compare their own daily practice with a model of practice description outlined within the College's framework of professional practice. This framework is comprised of different competency areas, which have been derived from an occupational analysis of roles within the pharmacy profession. This framework includes a key statement of purpose, the identification of key roles, activities and their associated performance indicators (see below)

---

**The Framework of Professional Practice (College of Pharmacists British Columbia, 1997)**

**Key purpose statement**

To assist individuals and groups to achieve desired health outcomes by providing current, rational, safe and cost effective pharmaceutical information, products and services

**Key roles**

1  PROVIDE PHARMACEUTICAL CARE
2  Produce, store, distribute and dispose of drug preparations
3  Contribute to the management of pharmacy practice

---

4 Maintain professional development and contribute to professional development of others

5 Contribute to the effectiveness of the health care system

**Activities (from Key Role 1)**
1 PROVIDE PHARMACEUTICAL CARE

A ASSESS THE CLIENT'S HEALTH STATUS AND NEEDS
B Develop a care plan with the client
C Implement the care plan

**Performance indicators (from Activity A)**
1 PROVIDE PHARMACEUTICAL CARE

A ASSESS THE CLIENT'S HEALTH STATUS AND NEEDS
1 Establish and maintain relationship with the client
   a) client is acknowledged promptly and effort is made to establish a relationship
   b) a safe, quiet and private environment is created, as feasible
   c) confidentiality is maintained
   d) client is encouraged to express his/her needs and views
   e) role, responsibilities and accessibility of the pharmacist in supporting the client is clarified and confirmed with the client.

- *professional portfolio assessment*: The professional portfolio provides a framework for practitioners to reflect upon and against which to record their professional and practice development activities. This enables pharmacists to assess and monitor their practice against the framework of professional practice.
- *knowledge assessment*: Multiple-choice questions are used to evaluate the practitioners' knowledge of medicines and their expected effects upon patients.
- *structured performance assessment*: This is an interactive tool which is used to assess a range of practice-related clinical skills and competences. Participants work through multiple stations performing tasks and responding to simulated patient problem scenarios.

The Continuing Assessment, Reflection and Enhancement (CARE) programme is being piloted throughout British Columbia as a model for mandatory re-licensure. The CARE programme encompasses many of the features of contemporary professional development programmes. These include the adoption of learner-centred approaches towards assessment and compilation of evidence, assessment of individuals against defined standards for practice, utilization of a wide evidence base to support claims for competence, adoption of a portfolio approach to facilitate reflection and link theory with practice, and the adoption of quality assurance mechanisms to validate the outcomes of assessment. These features are summarized in Figure 5.1. These principles appear to reflect a global education and training strategy for professionals, which is being developed in response to:

- the need for world-class standards, so that nations may remain competitive at a time when advances in telecommunications and information technologies are transforming delivery systems for education and training and learner support
- the development of world-class standards, which are now becoming a basis for the marketing of education and training programmes
- the need for international articulation, for example, leading nations such as Canada, the UK and the USA have been developing national standards for education and training in order to achieve wider acceptance of qualifications and credentials
- the need for portability and transferability of professional qualifications, to ensure that a common standard for practice has been achieved.

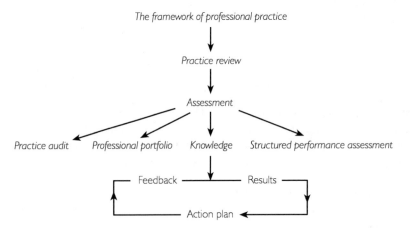

**Figure 5.1**   The CARE programme model (College of Pharmacists British Columbia, 1997)

## UK: University of Sheffield degree in Community Nursing

The Bachelor in Medical Science Honours degree in Specialist Community Nursing Practice is a modular programme of studies that leads to the award of a degree in Specialist Community Nursing, and a licensed specialist qualification with the statutory nursing body.

The programme develops knowledge and expertise by critically evaluating past experiences, gives students a broader understanding of the requirements for community care, increases the knowledge required to underpin community nursing practice and enables students to reflect on competencies in a specific area of community care.

The scheme is an important component of the ENB Framework for Continuing Professional Education, and supports this by ensuring that the ten key characteristics, believed to be common to all aspects of care delivery, are addressed within the professional knowledge base of the programme (Chapter 4).

The programme consists of five modules: reflective specialist community practice; research appreciation as applied to specialist community practice; education of clients, others; self-management and delivery of specialist community practice; and a dissertation module. Each module has specific learning outcomes which meet UKCC standards for education and practice that lead to each of the eight qualifications for specialist community practice.

Each module within the programme is assessed in theory and in practice. This approach towards assessment has become an important feature within the curriculum of the Nursing and Midwifery School, which has initiated a strategy which enables the student to achieve 'total competence', which is defined as:

> *the necessary skills, knowledge, attitudes, understanding and experience required in order to perform professional and occupational roles to a satisfactory standard within the workplace.*
>
> Day (1998)

The development of a complementary approach towards assessment of students within the School of Nursing and Midwifery meets the demands of managers who require fitness for purpose. Within the programme, a flexible approach towards assessment enables the student and the assessor to interpret the requirements of local care delivery according to the context in which professional care is delivered.

In planning the assessment strategy for the programme, it was realized that the current climate of fiscal restraint would require a different approach towards the assessment of students and the preparation and development of assessors. As a consequence, traditional methods for assessment of clinical competence, i.e. direct observation, were opened up to include more diverse activities, for example testimony from others.

As a result, assessors and students are now able to plan the time spent on assessment more appropriately by prioritizing evidence requirements according to the experience of the student, and the context in which they both work. This approach is particularly appropriate within the field of community nursing where practitioners often work autonomously, but report to a team for the purpose of case review. Therefore the recording of critical incidents by learning diary, or assessment by peers using a testimony, are the most cost-effective use of assessor time.

In this situation, the assessor is able to review the diverse evidence which has been generated by the student, adding to the evidence already collected by posing critical questions. As a result, feedback from assessors indicates that they are spending one and a half to two hours per week on assessment activities, a commitment which all assessors feel they are able to meet.

The rationale developed for the assessment strategy emphasizes the importance of 'total competence' so that the student is:

- *fit for purpose* – the requirements of employers
- *fit for practice* – the requirements of professional and statutory bodies
- *fit for award* – the academic requirements of the university.

Within this framework, there is considerable emphasis upon the collection of evidence that links theory with practice. This mechanism includes the development of a portfolio of evidence which requires students to complete a learning diary using the critical incident technique, and to complete practice-based evidence logs to record the processes and outcomes of assessment. These mechanisms provide valuable data for the students to draw upon when completing their theoretical assignments for each module.

Individuals accessing the programme have diverse academic and professional backgrounds. In order to accommodate this, a strategy for assessment of prior learning achievement has been developed in line with university and professional body regulations. The assessment strategy attempts to accommodate this by encouraging diverse methods of assessment, incorporating student self-assessment, and recognising witness testimony as possible evidence of competence.

The assessment strategy for the programme is student-led. Therefore all students are encouraged to undertake an assessment of their current competence. To do this, they are advised to refer to the clusters and descriptors that relate to the course and, working through each one, determine their level of competence using the scale shown below.

---

### Self-assessment scale

0 = I have no experience of this.
1 = I have observed or been orientated to this.
2 = I can participate and assist in this.
3 = I can do this with minimal supervision in a safe and competent manner.

---

The student records the outcome of their self-assessment, making notes of any particular task, responsibilities, projects or initiatives they have previously undertaken which enable them to demonstrate competence against the descriptor they are looking at. Low scores highlight areas on which the student needs to concentrate. High scores suggest areas where the student can already start to compile evidence.

After this period of self-assessment, the student is advised to meet with his or her personal tutor and assessor so that an assessment plan can be drawn up. The student is also advised to develop a personal profile by reflecting upon the following questions:

- What competencies do you think you already have?
- What areas of this module enable you to demonstrate existing competence?
- What are the competencies you need to develop in order to meet the requirements of the module?
- What are the plans you can agree to enable you to develop these competencies?

The competencies required of the student relate to the theoretical outcomes of the taught modules devised for the community programme. Each competency outcome consists of a *cluster statement* (key role) and a *descriptor* (activities relating to that key role). An example is shown below.

---

### Example of a cluster statement (key roles) and descriptors (activities)

1 Promotes equality for all individuals         *Cluster statement*
   a)   Promotes anti-discriminatory practice.
   b)   Promotes and supports client's rights and choice within health care delivery.
   c)   Acknowledges client's personal beliefs and identity.    *Descriptors*
   d)   Supports client's needs through effective communication.

---

Each competency outcome is founded on the underpinning *principles* outlined below.

---

### The principles underpinning key roles (clusters)

1 The evidence relating to each statement has been developed within a multi-cultural, multi-racial and multi-disciplinary environment.
2 The evidence presented demonstrates that the student has an understanding of the legal and ethical consequences of their action, and the implications this may have for professional practice.
3 The student is able to demonstrate an awareness of how contemporary research and policy issues may be applied to the community setting.
4 The assessment of client needs and health care delivery takes place within an holistic framework and an ethos of confidentiality.

---

Using these principles as a framework to underpin each cluster, the student is required to build up a portfolio of evidence which is presented to their assessor for assessment and to their verifier for verification. In order to achieve competence, the student must be able to demonstrate that each competency and its underlying principle has been achieved.

Whenever possible, evidence to support claims to competence is generated from activities undertaken by the student whilst under the direct supervision of an assessor. Where direct observation is inappropriate or inadvisable, the student and assessor may choose to utilize a different assessment method.

In order to elicit the relevant underpinning knowledge and understanding, direct observation is supplemented by other assessment methods. To facilitate this, the student is asked to keep a learning diary in order to justify his or her claim to 'knowing'. The diary is submitted by the student to the assessor as part of the assessment process, and is followed up by a question and answer session conducted by the assessor.

Throughout the assessment, emphasis is placed upon the need to *triangulate* evidence by ensuring that a range of assessment strategies is used by the assessor. The assessment method chosen by the student and assessor is recorded in the student's assessment plan. For example, in assessing the student's competence to take a client's health and social history, the assessor may choose to utilize the methods outlined in Figure 5.2.

The portfolio is the central focus for assessment activity within the programme. It put together the student's experience of clinical practice and how this relates to the theoretical components of the course. The portfolio also provides an opportunity for the student to reflect upon his or her practice in the community care environment. Each student is responsible for preparing and submitting the portfolio for assessment and verification at the end of each module. The personal tutor provides personal guidance on portfolio-building. The student is also given a handbook which contains the following information: definitions and guidelines for the development of a portfolio; guidelines for use of a learning diary, plus a learning diary *pro-forma*; how to conduct an initial self-assessment and a *pro-forma* for doing this; assessment of practice guidelines,

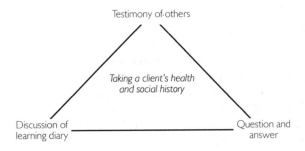

**Figure 5.2**   Triangulating evidence

with sample assessment plans and assessment records; a copy of the competencies to be achieved.

In developing a portfolio, students are required to support their claim to competence by generating a diverse range of evidence. This evidence must demonstrate that the learner has achieved the necessary professional, personal and occupational competencies, together with the relevant underpinning knowledge and understanding required for each module. At the end of each module, the verifier sees the portfolio. If it meets the requirements of the programme, it is approved and countersigned. Each portfolio is subject to inspection by the external examiner or the examination board. On completion of the programme, the learner keeps the portfolio as a record of competence for prospective employers, as a baseline for further development or to meet the mandatory continuing registration requirements of the statutory body.

The use of a portfolio to record both the process and product of a learner's competence has become an important feature within the nursing curriculum. This type of approach is consistent with recommendations laid down by the professional body, which identifies the need to clarify assessment outcomes, promote the use of portfolio approaches to assessment, and argues for a diverse evidence base in assessing the competence of a student.

## SUMMARY

The various methods which learners might use to generate evidence of prior learning have been discussed and presented, with particular emphasis being placed upon the need to:

- generate evidence that is relevant to any outcomes or competencies required
- carefully plan work and/or learning in order to maximize the evidence produced
- record evidence in a meaningful and constructive way, using a portfolio
- utilize evidence from diverse and various sources.

These issues are now summarized in the form of a checklist that the practitioner can use to review the evidence that the learner is presenting in his or her portfolio. The following questions highlight key issues to consider:

- Is the evidence relevant to the outcomes or competencies required?
- Does the evidence cover all of the criteria?
- Does the learner have the necessary supporting knowledge and understanding?
- Is the evidence up-to-date?
- Is the evidence real and not fabricated?
- Is the evidence the product of the learner's own work?
- Is the confidentiality of any sensitive information maintained?
- Is the evidence laid out in a clear and consistent way?
- Will the assessor be able to easily follow the evidence presented in the portfolio?

A portfolio enables adult learners to give a detailed account of their skills and abilities in relation to the outcomes and criteria being assessed. In order to do this it should:

- be structured in a clear and logical way
- be supported by evidence from others, e.g. colleagues, peers, supervisors, etc.
- describe the learner's learning and/or work environment and the daily activities in which he or she participates
- be easy to read and understand
- allow the learner some freedom of expression.

APL, as exemplified by the portfolio development process, enables adult learners to create valid, reliable and comprehensive documents based on their own unique strengths and life circumstances.

For many adults, the preparation of a portfolio affirms their self-worth, enhances their self-confidence and strengthens their capacity to pro-actively deal with the many transitions in their lives. A well-prepared portfolio also enables them to achieve formal credit and recognition for their skills and competencies.

The next chapter is designed to help you to develop your own portfolio, so that your continuing competence to practise can be affirmed and your personal development needs can be addressed.

# 6 LIFE-LONG LEARNING AND THE APL PRACTITIONER

This book has discussed the role of the APL practitioner and how emerging models of practice are influencing the role of the APL adviser and assessor. Within this book, the following issues have been discussed:

- adult learning theory and its relationship to APL
- the concept of APL and its benefit to students, employers and the professions
- the principles underpinning a credit-based system
- factors influencing the practice of assessment of prior learning
- the use of guidelines and benchmarks to clarify the APL practitioner's role
- the role of the APL adviser, assessor and co-ordinator
- factors which might influence the role of the APL practitioner
- the principles of rigorous assessment, e.g. validity, reliability, sufficiency, etc.
- developmental, credit-based and complementary models of APL practice
- the portfolio approach to APL.

More specifically, your attention has been drawn to the emergence of benchmarks for APL practice, and the ways in which these might influence your development as a practitioner (Appendix 1). Throughout this text, you have had an opportunity to engage in key learning activities and discussions. You may have followed these in a logical or sequential way, or you may have 'dipped' into a chapter or an activity as the need arose. Regardless of the reading strategy you have used, your experience of this book will have, undoubtedly, allowed you to generate a plethora of evidence, which will enable you to document and record your existing competence, as well as your continuing development, as an APL practitioner. This chapter examines further strategies which will enable you to do this.

At the end of this chapter, you will be able to:

- conduct a library search in order to identify appropriate literature relating to APL
- systematically read and review appropriate APL literature
- construct a card index system in order to record appropriate APL literature
- identify a personal strategy for continuous development of your role as an APL practitioner.

## ADULT LEARNING

As a younger person you were probably aware of how quickly you were able to develop and try out new ideas, often at an alarming rate. Unfortunately, as an individual matures, the capacity to learn so much information often diminishes. The adult learner can overcome this by drawing upon his or her vast knowledge and experience of life. Any new learning becomes easier if it is made interesting and relevant – particularly if it is related to the world of work!

The adult learner needs to try out ideas, test them and apply them to his or her everyday experience before they can be retained. How individuals do this varies, some might take immediate action and then reflect upon their experience; others might think carefully and plan a strategy before they act. Whatever the starting point, research into adult learning has shown that mature students often move through a common cycle of learning (see Figure 6.1).

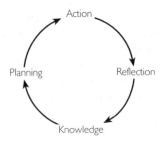

**Figure 6.1** The adult learning cycle

In practice, it would be more realistic to view this process as a *spiral* rather than a circle – as learning never ceases, with each new skill or piece of knowledge we acquire enabling us to plan ahead, giving us something to draw upon when encountering new problems or situations. Much of the time we are not conscious of moving through this process. However, if we stop to think about it, we would probably be aware of having learned from some previous experience.

## DEVELOPING YOUR OWN PORTFOLIO

When compiling a portfolio of evidence, you are going through this process in a more self-aware and reflective way. For example, your portfolio and the items in it mean you have thought about:

- what you are trying to do
- the most effective way of doing this
- what you need to know in order to do this
- how well you are succeeding
- why one particular approach to APL works ... but not another
- what you would do differently next time.

Your experience with this book has engaged you in an active process which has encouraged you to continually seek out new information and apply it to your working practice, which you can then document in your own portfolio using a learning diary (Appendix 2). It is the process of *seeking out* and *applying* information that this chapter will now cover.

## USING A LIBRARY

The library is an essential resource for those who are undertaking an APL practitioner role. Use of the library will help you to gather relevant information and will also provide you with a quiet and peaceful environment in which you can study – quite a luxury for those of us who lead busy lives!

You may be fortunate in having easy access to your college or university library, or alternatively you will have access to the local authority library service. If you are not already a member of a library, it will be in your interest to join one. However, be careful to select one that will offer services and resources to suit your needs – not all libraries provide specialist advice on APL, and some may charge you for accessing this type of information. Most libraries will offer the following:

- books on long- and short-term loan
- periodicals and journals
- bibliographies: a list of publications, historical and current
- inter-library loans
- government publications
- dictionaries
- audio-visual equipment, e.g. pre-recorded video or audio tapes
- computer search facilities using CD-ROM
- photographic and photocopying services.

All library information is catalogued in a systematic way whether it is books, journals, newspapers, etc. Accessing this stored information might appear complex, but libraries have organized and developed systems that can be used to do this.

### Manual storage systems

The *Dewey system* is most commonly used for categorizing books stored in the library. It is a system that allocates three-figure numbers to each category of books within a library. For example, 000 refers to *Generalities*, 100 refers to *Philosophy and related disciplines*, 200 refers to *Religion*, and so on.

Many of these categories are so large that the category number is then broken down into parts or sub-sets of that number. This makes their storage and retrieval easier. For example, 800 refers to *Literature*, but *American Literature in English* is categorized as 810, whilst *English and Anglo-Saxon Literature* is classified as 820, etc. (You are familiar with this type of arrangement in NVQs where units are broken down into elements, and then finally into performance criteria – Chapter 1.)

To use the Dewey system, you need to access the library's card index. You can either look up information under the subject title or the author's surname. On the card that corresponds to the book you are looking for you will find the Dewey number. You can then use this number to locate the the book on the library shelves. Many libraries also store this information on microfiche film which you access using a microfiche reader.

Visit your local library and familiarize yourself with the Dewey numbers associated with your subject area. Remember you are looking at general categories such as *Education and training* or *Adult continuing education*. It is from these general categories that you might find the specific subject of *Assessment of prior learning*. The librarian will be able to assist you with this activity

## Computerized storage systems

You can use computers to help you locate a journal article or a book relating to the subject you are currently studying. You can do this by using:

- *CD-ROMs* – for research and journal articles
- the *On-line Public Access Catalogue* (OPAC) – for books
- the *Internet*.

## CD-ROMs

You can use specialized CD-ROMs to search for information using a personal computer. This is a very powerful and quick way of identifying the information you require. One of the most useful CD-ROMs is the British Education Index (BEI) or the American equivalent, ERIC.

Most libraries that use CD-ROMs will provide you with training and step-by-step advice on how to use the disk and the computer. To use a CD-ROM you insert the disk into the computer disk drive, press the appropriate command key(s) to load the disk onto the computer, and then follow the commands on the screen.

Once loaded, the computer will ask you to enter your search terms (*key words*) – you will need to be clear and succinct about what it is you are searching for. You can do this by identifying words that you think will be used in the title of an article. For example, if you are searching for information about APL, remember the many acronyms that are used within different countries, e.g. APL, PLA, PLAR, RPL. Remember also that words such as *the* or *of* will throw up several thousand sources of information, as these words are used in the title of many journal articles. To overcome this, you need to refine and limit the key words you are searching for. It is suggested that you do this before you use ERIC – to avoid getting side-tracked!

Once you have located the information you require, you can instruct the computer to print it (the hard copy). You can then use this hard copy as a reference to help you retrieve any of the articles you have identified.

## OPAC

OPAC helps you to identify the location of books in the library. It has an author and subject index, plus a facility to enter key words, which will help you to search in a more accurate way for the information you require.

## The Internet

Many journals now have on-line archives, from which relevant articles can be searched and retrieved via a personal computer, provided the computer is appropriately programmed and is connected to the Internet via a modem. In addition there may be useful practitioner information which can be obtained from world wide websites. For example, some useful sites for APL include:

- Canada: http://nall.oise.utoronto.ca
- UK: http://www.seec-office.org.uk
- USA: http://www.cael.org/
- South Africa: http://www.el.uct.ac.za/rpl/

NB Punctuation for these website addresses is critical.

## Other sources of information

As an APL practitioner you will want to read articles relating to adult learning and assessment either from journals, magazines or newspapers (see *Recommended further reading*, page 96). At times you may need to review several articles either from different sources or across a period of time. If the articles are not available in your local library, they may be obtained through inter-library loan (some libraries may charge for this). Alternatively, they can be obtained from on-line archives, using the Internet.

## READING

Visiting a library is often an enjoyable experience. However, the task of reading requires some organization. You are not expected to read everything written about a single topic, therefore it is very important that you establish which book or article is the most important to read.

You will find that people adopt different strategies for reading, so it is important that you identify your own needs. It is useful to begin by asking:

- Why am I reading this book or article?
- How is it relevant?
- What am I getting from it that is new to me?

### Getting started

Here is a simple method of making the best of your reading. It is known as the SQ3R method, which stands for: *survey, question, read, recall and review* (Williams, 1989).

### Survey
- For a book, scan its contents page and its index to see what you can expect to get out of it.

- For an article, scan the abstract, introduction and summary.

Take note of headings, sub-headings, bold print and italics. Read the first sentence of each paragraph – this type of reading will help you to gain an overview of the content.

### Question
Identify questions you will be able to answer once you have read the book or article in more detail. The survey you have just completed will assist you in formulating the questions.

### Read
Having completed the above, read carefully and find the answers to your questions. There is little point in reading the remainder of the book or article. End of chapter summaries may help you to carry out this activity.

### Recall
Try to answer all your questions without looking at the book or your notes. This way you will realize what you have learned and what you need to concentrate on.

### Review
To check the accuracy of the information you have gained, read the relevant sections in the book or article again.

## Effective reading
Effective reading is not associated with how fast you can read, but it is about being flexible and purposeful. There are, however, techniques that can enhance your reading skills and your learning. For example:

- Identify the purpose for the reading – don't get side-tracked!
- Seek out the relevant, and therefore the most important, information.
- Evaluate the content for its relevance to your prior knowledge.
- At intervals break off to reflect on your understanding of the content.
- Make a conscious effort to interpret the text and draw conclusions.
- Make brief notes to aide your memory.

In making your notes, add your own comments and evaluations. Get into the habit of writing summaries and compare these with the summaries your colleagues have written. Make sure you record the source of your information by noting the author, date of publication, journal or book title, etc. For example:

- For a book:
  a) Challis, M. (1993). *Introducing APEL.* Routledge, London.

b) Blower, D. (2000). Canada: The story of prior learning assessment and recognition *in* Evans, N. (ed.). *Experiential Learning Around the World: Employability and the Global Economy*. Jessica Kingsley, London. ISBN 185302736 7.

- For a journal article:
  Butterworth, C. (1992). More than one bite at the APEL: contrasting models of accrediting prior learning. *Journal of Further and Higher Education*. Vol. 16, No. 3, pp 39-51.

NB Book and journal titles are usually printed in italic type. If you are handwriting the titles, underline them instead.

## Maintaining a card index system

It is suggested that you record the information you gain from your reading on index cards. These can be stored in a box with alphabetical dividers, or alternatively stored as files within a folder on floppy disk or on the hard drive of your computer. The information recorded should include:

- details of the book or article
- how it fits in to your area of study
- any useful quotes: use inverted commas to show that they are quoted, note the page number
- a brief summary of the article: a CD-ROM print-out could be useful here
- your own evaluation of the article
- any further sources of information the article may refer too.

The style you use is up to you, but be consistent with your approach.

## Organising your card index system

It will be useful to organize your information under the categories you wish to study. For example, the following headings might be useful to you as an APL practitioner:

1 Adult learning
2 Assessment methods
3 APL policy and procedure
4 The role of the APL practitioner.

It is also useful to keep every item of information on a separate card, or within a separate file on your computer so that it can be assembled in a variety of ways – if information you have read is of value in relation to several categories, it will then be easier to cross-reference your reading. For example, you may want to reference the CAPLA publication *Developing Benchmarks for Assessment of Prior Learning* under sections two, three and four of your index (see above). This may sound a laborious task, but it will be worth it in the long run, particularly when you are identifying evidence towards an APL practitioner credential!

## SUMMARY

This chapter has focused on adult learning, study skills, the use of library facilities and the different methods of searching for information. Various methods for effective reading and recording of information have also been discussed, and a mechanism for indexing appropriate literature has been suggested. If you have worked through this chapter, you will be able to use the library and organize your reading material in a more meaningful way, so that you can successfully meet the 'underpinning' knowledge requirements of your APL practitioner role.

Learning never stops, it is a constant feature of adult life. To assist you, a short list of recommended reading on APL is included on page 96.

# REFERENCES

American Council on Education (2001). *Bridges of Opportunity: A History of the Center for Adult Learning and Educational Credentials*. American Council on Education, Washington, DC.

Anderson, B. (1998). The management leadership challenges: are the teachers and administrators ready to become the learners? *Joint Education Trust Bulletin*. 6–7.

Barr, R.B. and Tagg, J. (1995). From teaching to learning: a new paradigm for undergraduate education. *Change*. 27 (6), pp 12–25.

Bernstein, B. (1996). *Pedagogy, Symbolic Control and Identity: Theory, Research, Critique*. Sage, Thousand Oaks.

Blower, D. (2000). Canada: the story of assessment of prior learning and recognition *in* Evans, N. (ed.). *Experiential Learning Around the World: Employability and the Global Economy*. Jessica Kingsley, London. ISBN 1-8530-2736-7.

Brown, S., Race, P. and Smith, B. (1996). *500 Tips on Assessment*. Kogan Page, London.

Butterworth, C. (1992). More than one bite at the APEL: contrasting models of accrediting prior learning. *Journal of Further and Higher Education*. Vol. 16, No. 3, pp 39–51.

Care Sector Consortium (1992). *National Occupational Standards for Care*. HMSO, London.

CAEL/APQC (1999). *Best Practices in Adult Learning*. Kendall/Hunt, Dubuque, Ohio. ISBN 0-8281-1429-3.

Challis, M. (1993). *Introducing APEL*. Routledge, London.

Clarke, M.C. (1993). Transformational learning. *New Directions for Adult and Continuing Education*. 57, pp 47–56.

College of Pharmacists British Columbia (1997). Continuing Assessment, Reflexion and Enhancement (RxCARE). Pilot program: a model for continuing competence assurance.

Committee of University Principals (CUP) (1987). *Macro-aspects of the University within the Context of Tertiary Education in the Republic of South Africa*. CUP, Pretoria.

Council for South African Trade Unions (1999). *Recognition of Prior Learning Guidelines Report*. COSATU, Pretoria.

Council for South African Trade Unions (2000). *Employment Equity: A South African German Cooperation*. COSATU, Pretoria.

Craft, W., Evans, N. and Keeton, M. (1997). *Learners All – Worldwide: A Dissemination Document*. Learning from Experience Trust, Chelmsford, UK.

Cross, K.P. (1994). The coming of age of experiential education. *National Society for Experiential Education Quarterly*. Vol. 19, No. 3, 1, pp 22–4.

Daloz, L.A. (1986) *Effective Teaching and Mentoring: Realizing the Transformational Power of Adult Learning Experiences*. Jossey-Bass, San Francisco.

Day, M, (1991). Accreditation of learning experience. *Nursing*. Vol. 4, No. 25, pp 35–236.

Day, M. (1996) *The Role of the Assessor: NVQs and the 'D' Units*. Nelson Thornes, Cheltenham, UK.

Day, M. (1998). Community education: a portfolio approach. *Nursing Standard*. Vol. 13, No. 10, pp 40–4.

Day, M. (2000). *Developing Benchmarks for Assessment of Prior Learning and Recognition: Practitioner Perspectives*. Canadian Association for Assessment of Prior Learning, Ontario, Canada.

Day, M. (2001). Developing benchmarks for assessment of prior learning. Part 1: research. *Nursing Standard*. Vol. 15, No. 34, pp 37–44.

Day, M. and Zakos, P. (1999). *Guidelines for the Validation of Competencies against the Canadian Technology Standards. Part II: For Validating Agents*. Canadian Technology Human Resources Board, Ottawa, Ontario. ISBN 0-9684-0076-0.

Evans, N. (ed.) (2000). *Experiential Learning Around the World: Employability and the Global Economy*. Jessica Kingsley, London. ISBN 1-8530-2736-7.

Flowers, R. and Hawke, G. (2000). The recognition of prior learning in Australia *in* Evans, N. (ed.). *Experiential Learning Around the World: Employability and the Global Economy*. Jessica Kingsley, London. ISBN 1-8530-2736-7

Gamson, Z.F. (1989). *Higher Education and the Real World: The Story of CAEL*. Longwood Academic, Wolfeboro, NH.

Harris, J. (1997) *Recognition of Prior Learning (RPL): Introducing a Conceptual Framework*. Cape Town University Press.

Harris, J. (2000). *RPL: Power, Pedagogy and Possibility*. Human Sciences Research Council, Pretoria, South Africa. ISBN 0-7969-1965-8.

Higher Education Quality Council (1994). *Choosing to Change. Extending access, choice and mobility in higher education*. The report of the HEQC CAT Development Project. HEQC. ISBN 1-8582-4150-2

Kasworm, C.E. and Marienau, A. (1997). Principles for assessment of adult learning. *New Directions for Adult and Continuing Education*. No. 75, Fall 1997. Jossey-Bass, San Francisco.

Keeton, M.T. (2000). Recognizing learning outside of schools in the United States of America *in* Evans, N. (ed.). *Experiential Learning Around the World: Employability and the Global Ecconomy*. Jessica Kingsley, London. ISBN 1-8530-2736-7

Keeton, M. (1999). Assessing and credentialing learning from prior experience *in* Messick, S. (ed.). *Assessment in Higher Education: Issues of Access, Quality, Student Development and Public Policy: A Festschrift in Honor of Warren W. Willingham* (pp 47–55). Erlbaum, Mahwah, NJ.

Khanyile, T. (2000). Recognition of prior learning its relevance to the proposed unified model of education and training for South African nurses. *Curationis*, 23 (2), pp 70–5.

Kolb, D.A. (1984) *Experiential Learning*. Prentice Hall, Englewood Cliffs, NJ.

Knowles, M.S. (1980). *The Modern Practice of Adult Education*. Association Press, Chicago.

Lewis, L.H. and Williams, C.J. (1994). Experiential learning: past and present, *in* Jackson, L. and Caffarella, R.S. (eds). *Experiential Learning: A New Approach*. Jossey-Bass, San Francisco. *New Directions for Adult and Continuing Education*. 62, pp 5–16.

Maehl, W.H. (2000). *Lifelong Learning at its Best: Innovative Practices in Adult Credit Programs*. Jossey-Bass, San Francisco.

Mann, C.M. (1998). *Credit for Lifelong Learning*, 5th edition. Bloomington. *In* Tichenor ISBN 4-00031-069-0.

McCrory, R. (1992). *Understanding National Vocational Qualifications and Standards: A Handbook*. Parthenon, Lancs.

McMillan, J. (1997). *Access Learning and Contexts: Issues and Implications (for RPL)*.

Paper commissioned for HSRC/UCT/Peninsula Technikon Research and Development Program in RPL.

Merriam, S.B. and Caffarella, R.S. (1999). *Learning in Adulthood: A Comprehensive Guide*, 2nd edition. Jossey-Bass, San Francisco.

Merrifield, J. *et al.* (2000). *Mapping APEL: Accreditation of Prior Experiential Learning in English Higher Education.* Learning from Experience Trust, Goldsmiths College, London.

Mezirow, J. (1991) *Transformative Dimensions of Adult Learning.* Jossey-Bass, San Francisco.

Michelson, E. (2001). Social transformation and the assessment of prior learning. *CAEL Forum News.* 24 (3), pp 28–31.

National Center for Education Statistics (1997) *Non-traditional Undergraduates: Trends in Enrolment from 1981 to 1992 and Persistence and Attainment among 1989–90 Beginning Post-secondary Students* (Statistical Analysis Report DEd, OERI Publication No. NCES 97-578). US Government Printing Office, Washington, DC.

National Commission on Higher Education (1997). Report Document. Department of Education, Pretoria.

National Council for Vocational Qualifications (1989). *National Vocational Qualifications: Criteria and Procedures.* NCVQ, London.

National University Continuing Education Association (1990). *Lifelong Learning Trends.* Author, Washington, DC.

O'Banion, T. (1997). *A Learning College for the 21st Century.* American Council on Education and Oryx Press, Phoenix.

Paczuska, A. and Randall, J. (1996). Using learning from work for progression to higher education: a degree of experience. *Journal of Vocational Education and Training.* Vol. 48, No. 4, pp 385–92.

Quality Assurance Agency for Higher Education (2000). *Code of Practice for the Assurance of Academic Quality and Standards in Higher Education. Section 6: Assessment of Students.* May 2000. QAA.

Ralph, A. (2000). *Assessor Training: Lessons from the Evaluation of an industry Based Training Course.* Council of Higher Education Report. Joint Education Trust, Gauteng.

Rogers, R.C. (1969). *Freedom to Learn.* Columbus, Ohio.

Rose, A.D. (1989). Non traditional education and the assessment of prior learning *in* Merriam, S.B. and Cunningham, P.M. (eds). *Handbook for Adult and Continuing Education* (pp 211–20). Jossey-Bass, San Francisco.

Rowley D.J., Lyan, H.D. and Dolence, M.G. (1998). *Strategic Choices for the Academy: How Demand for Lifelong Learning will Recreate Higher Education.* Jossey-Bass, San Francisco.

Rowntree, D. (1987). *Assessing Students. How Shall We Know Them?* Kogan Page, London.

SEEC (undated). *Credit accumulation and transfer* (online). Southern England Consortium for Credit Accumulation and Transfer. http://www.seec-office.org.uk/credit.html (accessed 9 January 2001).

SEEC (1995). *A Quality Code for AP(E)L Issues for Managers and Practitioners.* Proceedings of the SEEC National Conference. 6 December 1995. Regents College, London. Southern England Consortium for Credit Accumulation and Transfer.

Sheckley, B.G. and Keeton, M.T. (1994; Fall/Winter, 1995). Assessing prior learning: educational benefits. *CAEL Forum and News*, Vol. 18, No. 1, pp 9–12.

Simosko, S. (1992) *Get Qualifications for What You Know and Can Do: A Personal Guide to APL*. Kogan Page, London. ISBN 0-7494-0475-2.

Tanner, D. and Tanner, L.N. (1980). *Curriculum Development: Theory into Practice.* Macmillan, New York.

Tate, P. (1999, January). *Levers for Change in Workforce Development Systems.* Paper presented at the League for Innovation Conference, New Orleans.

Tough, A.M. (1967). *Learning Without a Teacher: A Study of Tasks and Assistance During Adult Self-Teaching Projects.* Ontario Institute for Studies in Education, Toronto, Ontario.

Training and Development Lead Body (1995). *National Standards for Training and Development*. Employment Department Group, Sheffield. ISBN 0 86392 4441.

Trowler, P. (1996). Angels in marble? Accrediting prior experiential learning in higher education. *Studies in Higher Education*. Vol. 21, No. 1, pp 17–30.

UCAS (1996). *Accreditation of Prior Learning*. UCAS Survey. http://www.ucas.ac.uk/higher/candq/apl/survey/index.html (accessed 8 November 2000).

Usher, R. and Edwards, R. (1995). Confessing all? A postmodern guide to the guidance and counselling of adult learners. *Studies in the Higher Education of Adults*.

Vavi, Z. (2000). *COSATU RPL Guidelines*. COSATU, Pretoria.

Whitaker, U.G. (1989). *Assessing Learning: Standards, Principles and Procedures*. Council for Adult and Experiential Learning, Philadelphia.

Whitaker, U.G. (1994). CAEL at twenty: looking ahead. *National Society for Experiential Education Quarterly*. Vol. 19, No. 3, 8–9, p. 26.

Williams, K. (1989). *Study Skills*. Macmillan, London.

Willingham, W.W. (1977). *Principles of Good Practice in Assessing Experiental Learning*. Council for Adult and Experiential Learning, Columbia, MD.

Zucker, B.J., Johnson, C.C. and Flint, T.A. (1999). *Assessment of Prior Learning: A Guidebook to American Institutional Practices*. Kendall/Hunt, Dubuque, IA.

## RECOMMENDED FURTHER READING

Challis, M. (1993). *Introducing APEL*, Routledge, London.

Evans, N. (ed.) (2000). *Experiential Learning Around the World: Employability and the Global Economy*. Jessica Kingsley, London. ISBN 1-8530-2736-7.

Harris, J. (2000). *RPL: Power, Pedagogy and Possibility*. Human Sciences Research Council, Pretoria, South Africa. ISBN 0-7969-1965-8.

Mann, C.M. (1998). *Credit for Lifelong Learning*, 5th edition. Bloomington. *In* Tichenor, ISBN 4-0003-1069-0.

Nyatanga, L., Forman, D. and Fox, J. (1998). *Good practice in the Accreditation of Prior Learning*. Cassell, London. ISBN 0-3043-4650-0.

Simosko, S. (1992), *Get Qualifications for What You Know and Can Do: A Personal Guide to APL*. Kogan Page, London. ISBN 0-7494-0475-2.

# Appendix 1

Benchmarks for the assessment of prior learning

## Function 1: prepare the individual for assessment

### Activity I: help the individual to identify relevant learning
a) The individual is given clear and accurate information about the reasons for, and methods of, collecting and presenting evidence of prior learning.
b) The individual is encouraged to review all relevant and appropriate experience.
c) Outcomes or agreed-upon criteria which the individual may currently be able to achieve are accurately identified from a review of their experience.
d) The way in which support is given encourages self-confidence and self-esteem in the individual.
e) If the individual expresses disagreement with the advice offered possible alternatives are explained in a clear and constructive manner.

### Activity II: agree to and review an action plan for demonstration of prior learning
a) The individual is given accurate advice and appropriate encouragement to enable him or her to form realistic expectations of the value of his or her prior learning.
b) Any outcomes or agreed-upon criteria to be achieved are appropriate to the individual's prior learning and future aspirations.
c) Advice to the individual accurately identifies outcomes or agreed-upon criteria which might reasonably be claimed on the basis of prior learning.
d) Opportunities to use evidence from prior learning are accurately analyzed.
e) The individual plan agreed to identifies realistic targets to collect and present evidence of prior learning as efficiently as possible.
f) The individual's motivation and self-confidence is encouraged throughout.
g) If there is disagreement with the advice given, options available to the individual are examined clearly and constructively.
h) The plan is reviewed appropriately with the individual.

### Activity III: help the individual to prepare and present evidence for assessment
a) The individual is provided with suitable support to prepare a portfolio or other appropriate forms of evidence.
b) Guidance provided to the individual during evidence preparation encourages the efficient development of clear, structured evidence relevant to the outcomes or agreed-upon criteria being claimed.
c) Liaison with potential assessors establishes mutually convenient arrange-

ments for review of portfolio or evidence and maintains the individual's confidence.

d) Opportunities are identified for the individual to demonstrate outcomes or agreed-upon criteria where evidence from prior learning is not available.

e) Any institutional documentation, recording and procedural requirements are met.

f) If there is disagreement with the advice given, options available to the individual are examined clearly and constructively.

## Function 2: assess the individual

### Activity I: agree to and review an assessment plan

a) Any possible opportunities for collecting evidence are identified and evaluated for relevance against the outcomes or agreed-upon criteria to be assessed and their appropriateness to the individual's needs.

b) Evidence collection is planned to make effective use of time and resources.

c) The opportunities selected provide access to fair and reliable assessment.

d) The proposed assessment plan is discussed and agreed with the individual and others who may be affected.

e) If there is disagreement with the proposed assessment plan, options open to the individual are explained clearly and constructively.

f) The assessment plan specifies outcomes or agreed-upon criteria to be achieved, opportunities for efficient evidence collection, assessment methods and the timing of assessments.

g) Requirements to assure the authenticity, currency, reliability and sufficiency of evidence are identified.

h) Plans are reviewed and updated at agreed-upon times to reflect the individual's development.

### Activity II: judge evidence and provide feedback

a) Advice and encouragement to collect evidence efficiently is appropriate to the individual's needs.

b) Access to assessment is appropriate to the individual's needs.

c) The evidence is valid and can be attributed to the individual.

d) Only the agreed-upon criteria and/or outcomes are used to judge the evidence.

e) Evidence is judged accurately against all the relevant outcomes or agreed-upon criteria.

f) When evidence of prior learning is used, checks are made that the individual can currently achieve the relevant outcome or agreed-upon criteria.

g) Evidence is judged fairly and reliably.

h) Difficulties in authenticating and judging evidence are referred promptly to the appropriate person(s).

i) When evidence is not to the agreed standard, the individual is given a clear explanation and appropriate advice.

j)    Feedback following the decision is clear, constructive, meets the individual's needs and is appropriate to his/her level of confidence.

### Activity III: make an assessment decision using differing sources of evidence and provide feedback

a)    The decision is based on all of the relevant evidence available.

b)    Any inconsistencies in the evidence are clarified and resolved.

c)    When the combined evidence is sufficient to cover the outcomes or the agreed-upon criteria, the individual is informed of his/her achievement.

d)    When evidence is insufficient, the individual is given a clear explanation and appropriate advice.

e)    Feedback following the decision is clear, constructive, meets the individual's needs and is appropriate to his/her level of confidence.

f)    The individual is encouraged to seek clarification and advice.

g)    Evidence and assessment decisions are recorded to meet any audit requirements.

h)    Any documentation is legible and accurate, stored securely and referred promptly to the next appropriate stage of the recording/certification process.

adapted from TDLB (1995) and Day (2000)

**NQF**  National Qualifications Framework for South Africa.

**PLA**  Prior Learning Assessment, the term for APL which is used in the USA.

**Reliability**  The degree to which an assessor's opinion may match that of another assessor in the same situation, with the same learner, using the same criteria. Reliability can be improved if advisers and assessors are able to meet on a regular basis to discuss and agree assessment requirements in order to achieve some standardization and consistency of approach. This is an activity which is often overseen by the APL co-ordinator.

**RPL**  Recognition of Prior Learning, the South African term for APL.

**SAQA**  South African Qualifications Authority.

**SEEC**  UK-based CATs consortium of around 40 different universities, and an APL practitioner network, within the south east of England. Contact: www.seec-office.org

**Simulation**  An assessment method which is based on direct observation of any performance other than the learner's normal, naturally-occurring work activity. Simulation can be used as an assessment method if safety or confidentiality are an issue in the workplace. They may also be used if work placements for students are limited, e.g. use of demonstration workshops or clinical laboratories.

**Sufficiency**  If all of the criteria within each of the specified outcomes or competencies have been met then the evidence is said to be sufficient, e.g. the need to demonstrate both range and diversity of practice, or to demonstrate contingencies.

**Summative assessment**  Undertaken to judge a learner's knowledge, skills and values at a defined point in time for the purpose of awarding a final grade, or granting some credit.

**Triangulation**  The use of several (and different) assessment methods to cross-validate (or confirm) the performance and underpinning knowledge of a learner against the required competency or outcome.

**UCAS**  University Careers Advisory Service, a UK organization for higher education.

**Validity**  An assessment should only be based upon the required outcomes or competencies and their associated criteria. An assessment is said to be valid if the assessor refers only to these stated criteria. Validity can be improved if the assessment criteria are explicit and made clear to the adviser, assessor and the learner.

**Validation letter**  A letter from a knowledgeable and competent third party, which can be used to support an individual's claim to competence.

# FEEDBACK ON KEY LEARNING ACTIVITIES

## Introduction

Many of the responses to the key learning activities in each chapter will be individual or context-specific. However, it is important for those who are new to APL to have the benefit of some initial guidance (see below). Please feel free to contact the author at: m.r.day@sheffield.ac.uk to discuss your ideas and responses.

 ## Key Learning Activity 1, page 11

For example, Trowler (1996) identifies significant tensions underpinning practice, which include:

- *cultural*: equality versus elitism, particularly the concept of 'cultural capitalism' as a hidden criterion for access to higher education
- *educational*: education as a product versus education as a process (a similar debate is outlined by Butterworth [1992] in her definition of credit exchange versus developmental models for APL [see feedback on *Key learning activity 11*])
- *organizational*: the need to maintain quality to ensure fitness for purpose versus the effects of excessive surveillance on the learning process, in particular alienation rather than internalization of any learning derived through experience.

Each of these issues may impact upon the process, or may skew the assessment outcome. These tensions are also present, to some extent, within more traditional forms of assessment, e.g. see Day (1996: 31).

 ## Key learning activity 2, page 15

You might want to consider whether the policies you are reviewing are biased towards the institution. If so, what impact will this have on the APL process? Also, how transparent are the roles of the learner, and the APL adviser and APL assessor?

 ## Key learning activity 3, page 37

1  See Introduction and Chapter 1.
2  E.g. see Chapter 10 in Rogers, C.R. (1990). *Client Centred Therapy*. Redwood Burns, Wiltshire, ISBN 0-09457-990-1.

3   See Introduction and beginning of Chapter 1.
5   See Chapter 1, page 3.
6   See Chapter 1, page 7.
7   For example, see Trowler (1996).
8   See for example, stereotyping, experimenter effect, contrast effect. (Day 1996: 31).
9   See Chapter 1, page 6.
10  See Appendix 1 for key role, functions, activities and performance indicators.

## Key learning activity 4, page 39

2   For example, see pages 38–9.
3   For example, see Chapter 3, page 39.

## Key learning activity 9, page 53

You may wish to consider the following guidelines for documentation, which have been adapted from NCVQ (1989). Firstly, documentation must be auditable. Your co-ordinator needs to sample a percentage of all assessments undertaken by an assessor, and will therefore, need to trace any evidence generated by the learner. Auditors need to know where the evidence is, e.g. the shop floor, a filing cabinet or within a computer file, so that they can examine it for validity, sufficiency, authenticity, etc.

Secondly, the process of recording assessments must be consistent. Consistent assessment records will ensure that standardization of the assessment process is maintained. Thirdly, documents must be flexible enough to meet the diverse needs of organizations offering, and to cope with a variety of demands and circumstances. Fourthly, documentation must be simple and straightforward. Finally, documentation should be familiar to all learners. In addition, the design of the assessment records should reflect the following considerations:

1   *Economy*: Can the documentation be completed in an acceptable amount of time? Could recording time be reduced without affecting the assessment process? Is the system sustainable when an assessor has several learners to assess? Could outcomes be recorded on a group basis with learners, to reduce the workload? Could a learner take responsibility for recording some of his or her own assessment outcomes?
2   *Location*: Where will the assessment take place? Can the documents be used in all assessment situations? Can meetings or briefing sessions be used as assessment or review opportunities?
3   *People involved*: Could more than one assessor be used to carry out the assessment? Does the assessor have regular and direct contact with the learner? Does the assessor work in a different place to the learner? Is the

learner usually supervized? Will assessment affect the learner's daily work routine? Would any documentation place an unfair burden on the learner?

4   *The organization*: Could documentation be integrated with other organizational systems such as performance appraisal, training and development plans, or total quality management procedures?

## Key learning activity 10, page 70

1   See Chapter 1, page 7, and compare with the chosen case study.
2   See Chapter 1, page 6, and compare with the chosen case study.
3   For example in the case study chosen, has the role of the adviser and assessor been separated? Or are these functions taken on as a team or committee approach in order to reduce possible bias?
7   Within the US case study competencies are derived from the learners' experience. In the Canadian and UK case studies, competencies are devised by the professional body, i.e. the Canadian Technology Human Resources Board (CTHRB) and the United Kingdom Central Council for Nursing and Midwifery (UKCC).
8   In the US case study a developmental approach is used. This is client-centred and meets the individual needs of the adult learner. However this approach is often regarded as being abstract and highly subjective. In the UK case study, a credit exchange approach is used. Learners are required to meet the demands of an external validating body. The over-riding emphasis is on quality assurance and the objectivity of the assessment process in order to prove that the learner is 'fit for purpose'. In the Canadian case study, a complementary approach is used. The best principles from either approach are utilized to ensure that both the needs of the learner, and the demands of the external validating body, are met.

## Key learning activity 11, page 70

Butterworth (1992) indicates that two differing models for AP(E)L have been emerging since the 1970s. Firstly, the credit exchange model, this is used extensively within the UK National Vocational Qualifications framework. Secondly, the developmental model, this emphasizes the use of documentary evidence supported by reflective commentary. The developmental approach originated from the early work of CAEL in the USA.

Butterworth explains that within the credit exchange model the learner identifies areas of a programme that they have achieved, and then offers evidence of these past achievements. Credit is awarded if an assessor agrees that this evidence 'proves' possession of the necessary knowledge and abilities. The claimant exchanges proof of past achievements for course credits. Within this model significant interest is placed on accreditation of prior achievement. For example, within the NVQ system, a clear distinction is made between 'learning' as a process, and the output of such learning that is described as 'achievement'. Accreditation is based upon evidence of achievement, not learning.

Butterworth indicates that the developmental model emphasizes the critical importance of the reflective and transformatory phase of experiential learning. The initial stages of the developmental process are the same as those in the credit exchange model, that is, the learner identifies areas of the course they have already achieved, and begins to collate evidence to support their claim. However within the developmental model, Butterworth (1992) claims that acceptable evidence alone is not enough to justify the award of credit. There is, she argues, an additional element where the learner's reflection is supported by discussions with a tutor. The purpose of these discussions is to support the learner's personal and professional development. The assessor judges both the evidence and the reflective personal account before awarding appropriate credit.

Butterworth (1992) argues that within the developmental approach the learner has a significant additional component: a written or oral statement that reflects on his or her past experience, which clarifies the learning and professional development that has taken place.

Another significant element of the developmental model, Butterworth argues, is the dialogue between the learner and the counsellor or tutor, which helps to structure and focus the learner's reflection and evidence collection. This combination – dialogue with a supportive 'outsider' and the rigorous thinking necessary to move between a mere description of the experience to an analysis of the learning it led to – is key to the change process offered by the developmental model.

Some academics argue that the credit exchange model is limiting. For example, Trowler (1996) argues that it is reductionist and indicate that its origins are derived from a behavioural model of learning, therefore it has no place in higher-level learning. He further argues that although the credit exchange model can achieve an award of credit for the claimant, it is self-limiting, whereas the developmental model can achieve significant personal and professional development for the individual.

Butterworth (1992) agrees, she indicates that the developmental model is closely associated with the process of action research. The aim of action research is to develop a grounded theory that makes sense to practitioners. It is based on problems that practitioners identify. It involves them in data collection and interpretation and produces explanations and solutions that they can implement. Reflections encouraged within the developmental model can assist the learner to undertake an analysis of their own practice and to increase their professional expertise. Butterworth (1992) argues that this is a legitimate pedagogy for higher education.

# INDEX

Note: Abbreviations used in the index are: APL = assessment of prior learning; CAEL = Council for Adult and Experiential Learning; CLLP = Credit for Lifelong Learning Program; CTHRB = Canadian Technology Human Resources Board; SA = South Africa